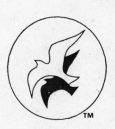

Published by
Rajneesh Foundation International
Rajneeshpuram, Oregon 97741 U.S.A.

# YOGA:

## THE SCIENCE OF THE SOUL

### VOLUME II

Discourses on the *Yoga Sutras* of Patanjali,
given at Shree Rajneesh Ashram, Poona, India
from January 1 to 10, 1975

## Bhagwan Shree Rajneesh

*Editor:* Swami Krishna Prabhu
*Design:* Swami Prem Deekshant
*Direction:* Ma Yoga Pratima, M.M., D.Phil. M. (RIMU), Arihanta
*Copyright:* 1976 Rajneesh Foundation International
*Published by:* Ma Anand Sheela, M.M., D.Phil.M.,
  D.Litt.M. (RIMU), Acharya
  Rajneesh Foundation International, President
  P.O. Box 9, Rajneeshpuram,
  Oregon 97741, U.S.A.

*First Edition:* (Entitled "Yoga: The Alpha and the Omega",
  Vol.2) 1976
*Second Edition:* July 1984 — 10,000 copies

Printed in U.S.A.

ISBN 0-88050-678-4
Library of Congress Catalog Number 84-42812

# Contents

# Contents

# Introduction

"Patanjali is the greatest scientist of the inner," says Bhagwan Shree Rajneesh. "He has a scientific mind, but his journey is inner. His terminology is that of a man who works in a scientific lab, but his lab is of the inner."

Five thousand years ago, in India, Patanjali set down his celebrated *Yoga Sutras*, a series of somewhat sparse, seed-like statements designed to guide seekers towards the same heights of consciousness he himself had attained. But to see the tree in the seed is no mean feat. Except for devoted disciples of yoga, Patanjali went pretty much unnoticed; no one had the insight or experience to understand just what he'd been talking about.

Five thousand years later, once more in India, the enlightened Master Bhagwan Shree Rajneesh gave a staggering one hundred ninety-minute discourses on Patanjali — and suddenly, what had been sparse became alive and juicy, what had been seeds blossomed into flowering trees.

YOGA: THE SCIENCE OF THE SOUL is not about twisting the body into strange-looking postures. It's about help. It's about practical, down-to-earth help for anyone interested in embarking on the most miraculous journey of scientific discovery ever — man's effort to move from his circumference to his center, to travel from his body inwards towards his soul.

In 1984, oddly enough, nothing seems more relevant than this unbeatable combination of Bhagwan Shree Rajneesh and Patanjali. This series is exactly for the present-day man, raised in an age of technology, with an understanding of the scientific approach, with an appreciation of the scientific mind. And, in particular, it is for the adventurous modern-day man who, surrounded by the crumbling structures and values of a world in chaos, has decided to take the responsibility for himself, has decided to explore, to evolve, to realize his own potential.

This volume is about a new brand of science, the science of religious experiment and inquiry, the science of attaining to one's own soul. Bhagwan Shree Rajneesh has merged the streams of science and religion. And he has created a rushing river — a river that overflows its banks to quench the thirst of anyone who comes near.

Swami Krishna Prem, M.M.,
D.Phil.M.(RIMU), Acharya

# Yoga:

## THE SCIENCE
## OF THE SOUL

### VOLUME II

Discourses on the *Yoga Sutras* of Patanjali,
given at Shree Rajneesh Ashram, Poona, India
from January 1 to 10, 1975

# The Meaning Of Samadhi

*Samprajnata samadhi is the samadhi that is accompanied by reasoning, reflection, bliss and a sense of pure being.*

*In asamprajnata samadhi there is a cessation of all mental activity, and the mind only retains unmanifested impressions.*

*Videhas and prakriti-layas attain asamprajnata samadhi because they ceased to identify themselves with their bodies in their previous life. They take rebirth because seeds of desire remained.*

*Others who attain asamprajnata samadhi attain through faith, effort, recollection, concentration and discrimination.*

P ATANJALI IS THE GREATEST scientist of the inner. His approach is that of a scientific mind: he is not a poet. And in that way he is very rare, because those who enter into the inner world are almost always poets, those who enter into the outer world are always almost scientists.

Patanjali is a rare flower. He has a scientific mind, but his journey is inner. That's why he became the first and the last word: he is the alpha and the omega. For five thousand years nobody could improve upon him. It seems he cannot be improved upon. He will remain the last word—because the very combination is impossible. To have a scientific attitude and to enter into the inner is almost an impossible possibility. He talks like a mathematician, a logician. He talks like Aristotle and he is a Heraclitus.

Try to understand his each word. It will be difficult: it will be difficult because his terms will be those of logic, reasoning, but his indication is towards love, towards ecstasy, towards God. His terminology is that of the man who works in a scientific lab, but his lab is of the inner being. So don't be misguided by his terminology, and retain the feeling that he is a mathematician of the ultimate poetry. He is a paradox, but he never uses paradoxical language. He cannot. He retains to the very firm logical background. He analyzes, dissects, but his aim is synthesis. He analyzes only to synthesize.

So always remember the goal—don't be misguided by the path—reaching to the ultimate through a scientific approach. That's why Patanjali has impressed the western mind very much. Patanjali has always been an influence. Wherever his name has reached, he has been an influence because you can understand him easily; but to understand him is not enough. To understand him is as easy as to understand an Einstein. He talks to the intellect, but his aim, his target, is the heart. This you have to remember.

We will be moving on a dangerous terrain. If you forget that he is a poet also, you will be misguided. Then you become too much attached to his terminology, language, reasoning, and you forget his goal. He wants you to go beyond reasoning, but *through* reasoning. That is a possibility. You can exhaust reasoning so deeply that you transcend. You go through reasoning; you don't avoid it. You use reason to go beyond it as a step. Now listen to his words. Each word has to be analyzed.

Samprajnata samadhi *is the* samadhi *that is*

*accompanied by reasoning, reflection, bliss and
a sense of pure being.*

He divides *samadhi*, the ultimate, in two steps. The ultimate cannot be divided. It is indivisible, and there are
no steps, in fact. But just to help the mind, the seeker, he
divides it first into two. The first step he calls *samprajnata samadhi*—a *samadhi* in which mind is retained in
its purity.

This first step, mind has to be refined and purified.
You simply cannot drop it, Patanjali says—it is impossible to drop it because impurities have a tendency to
cling. You can drop only when the mind is absolutely
pure—so refined, so subtle, that it has no tendency to
cling.

He does not say that "Drop the mind," as Zen Masters
say. He says that is impossible; you are talking nonsense. You are saying the truth, but that's not possible
because an impure mind has a weight. Like a stone, it
hangs. And an impure mind has desires—millions of
desires, unfulfilled, hankering to be fulfilled, asking to
be fulfilled, millions of thoughts incomplete in it. How
can you drop?—because the incomplete always tries to
be completed.

Remember, says Patanjali, you can drop a thing only
when it is complete. Have you watched? If you are a
painter and you are painting, unless the painting becomes complete you cannot forget it. It continues,
haunts you. You cannot sleep well; it is there. In the
mind it has an undercurrent. It moves; it asks to be
completed. Once it is completed, it is finished. You can
forget about it. Mind has a tendency towards comple-
tion. Mind is a perfectionist, and so whatsoever is
incomplete is a tension on the mind. Patanjali says you
cannot drop thinking unless thinking is so perfect that
now there is nothing to be done about it. You can simply drop it and forget.

This is completely the diametrically opposite way

from Zen, from Heraclitus. First *samadhi*, which is *samadhi* only for name's sake, is *samprajnata—samadhi* with a subtle purified mind. Second *samadhi* is *asamprajnata—samadhi* with no mind. But Patanjali says that when the mind disappears, then too there are no thoughts, then, too, subtle seeds of the past are retained by the unconscious.

The conscious mind is divided in two. First, *samprajnata*—mind with purified state, just like purified butter. It has a beauty of its own, but it is there. And howsoever beautiful, mind is ugly. Howsoever pure and silent, the very phenomenon of mind is impure. You cannot purify a poison. It remains poison. On the contrary, the more you purify it, the more poisonous it becomes. It may look very, very beautiful. It may have its own color, shades, but it is still impure.

First you purify; then you drop. But then too the journey is not complete because this is all in the conscious mind. What you will do with the unconscious? Just behind the layers of the conscious mind is a vast continent of unconscious. There are seeds of all your past lives in the unconscious.

Then Patanjali divides the unconscious into two. He says *sabeej samadhi*—when the unconscious is there and mind has been dropped consciously, it is a *samadhi* with seeds—*sabeej*. When those seeds are also burned, then you attain the perfect—the *nirbeej samadhi: samadhi* without seeds.

So conscious into two steps, then unconscious into two steps. And when *nirbeej samadhi*, the ultimate ecstasy, without any seeds within you to sprout and to flower and to take you on further journeys into existence. . .then you disappear.

In these sutras he says,

Samprajnata samadhi *is the* samadhi *that is accompanied by reasoning, reflection, bliss and a sense of pure being.*

But this is the first step; many are misguided—they think this is the last because it is so pure and you feel so blissful and so happy that you think that now nothing is there to be achieved more. If you ask Patanjali, he will say the *satori* of the Zen is just the first *samadhi*. It is not the final, the ultimate; ultimate is still far away.

The words that he uses cannot be exactly translated into English because Sanskrit is the most perfect language; no language comes even near to it. So I would have to explain to you. The word used is *vitarka*: in English it is translated as reasoning. It is a poor translation. *Vitarka* has to be understood. *Tarka* means logic, reasoning: then Patanjali says there are three types of logic. One he calls *kutarka*—reasoning oriented towards the negative: always thinking in terms of no, denying, doubting, nihilistic.

Whatsoever you say, the man who lives in *kutarka*—negative logic—always thinks how to deny it, how to say no to it. He looks to the negative. He is always complaining, grumbling. He always feels that something somewhere is wrong—always! You cannot put him right because this is his orientation. If you tell him to see to the sun, he will not see the sun. He will see the sunspots; he will always find the darker side of things: that is *kutarka*. That is *kutarka*—wrong reasoning—but it looks like reasoning.

It leads finally to atheism. Then you deny God, because if you cannot see the good, you cannot see the lighter side of life, how can you see God? You simply deny. Then the whole existence becomes dark. Then everything is wrong, and you can create a hell around you. If everything is wrong, how can you be happy? And it is your creation, and you can always find something wrong because life consists of a duality.

In the rose bush there are beautiful flowers, but thorns also. A man of *kutarka* will count the thorns, and then he will come to an understanding that this rose must be illusory; it cannot exist. Amidst so many thorns, millions of thorns, how can a rose exist? It is impossible; very possibility is denied. Somebody is deceiving.

Mulla Nasruddin was very, very sad. He went to the priest and said, "What to do? My crop is destroyed again. No rains." The priest said, "Don't be so sad, Nasruddin. Look at the lighter side of life. You can be happy because still you have much. And always believe in God who is the provider. He even provides for birds of the air, so why you are worried?" Nasruddin said, "Yes!" very bitterly, "Off my corn! God provides the birds of the air off my corn."

He cannot see the point. His crop is destroyed by these birds, and God is providing them. . ."and my crop is destroyed." This type of mind will always find something or other, and he will be always tense. Anxiety will follow him like a shadow. This Patanjali calls *kutarka* —negative logic, negative reasoning.

Then there is *tarka*—simple reasoning. Simple reasoning leads nowhere. It is moving in a circle because it has no goal. You can go on reasoning and reasoning and reasoning, but you will not come to any conclusion because reasoning can come to a conclusion only when there is a goal from the very beginning. You are moving in a direction, then you reach somewhere. If you move in all directions—sometimes to the south, sometimes to the east, sometimes to the west—you waste energy.

Reasoning without a goal is called *tarka*; reasoning with a negative attitude is called *kutarka*; reasoning with a positive grounding is called *vitarka*. *Vitarka* means special reasoning. So *vitarka* is the first element of *samprajnata samadhi*. A man who wants to attain to the inner peace has to be trained into *vitarka*—special reasoning. He always looks to the lighter side, the positive. He counts the flowers and forgets the thorns—not that there are not thorns, but he is not concerned with them. If you love the flowers and count the flowers, a moment comes when you cannot believe in the thorns, because how is it possible where so beautiful flowers exist, how can thorns exist? There must be something illusory.

The man of *kutarka* counts thorns; then flowers become illusory. The man of *vitarka* counts flowers; then thorns become illusory. That's why Patanjali says: *vitarka* is the first element. Only then bliss is possible. Through *vitarka* one attains to heaven. One creates one's own heaven all around.

Your standpoint counts. Whatsoever you found around you is your own creation—heaven or hell. And Patanjali says you can go beyond logic and reasoning only through the positive reasoning. Through the negative you can never go beyond, because the more you say no, the more you found things to be sad—no, denied. Then, by and by, you become a constant no inside—a dark night, only thorns and no flowers can flower in you—a desert. . .

When you say yes, you find more and more things to be said yes. When you say yes, you become a yea-sayer. Life is affirmed, and you absorb through your yes all that is good, beautiful, all that is true. "Yes" becomes the door in you for the divine to enter; "no" becomes a closed door. Door closed, you are a hell: doors open, all doors open, existence flows in you. You are fresh, young, alive; you become a flower.

*Vitarka, vichar, ananda:* Patanjali says if you are attuned with *vitarka*—a positive reasoning—then you can be a thinker, never before it. Then thinking arises. He has a very different meaning of thinking. You also think that you think. Patanjali will not agree. He says you have thoughts, but no thinking. That's why I say it is difficult to translate him.

He says you have thoughts, vagrant thoughts like a crowd, but no thinking. Between your two thoughts there is no inner current. They are uprooted things; there is no inner planning. Your thinking is a chaos. It is not a cosmos; it has no inner discipline. It is just like you see a rosary. There are beads; they are held together by an invisible thread running through them. Thoughts are beads; thinking is the thread. You have beads—too many, in fact, more than you need—but no inner running thread through them. That inner thread is called by Patanjali thinking—*vichar.* You have thoughts, but no thinking. And if this goes on and on, you will become mad. A madman is a man who has millions of thoughts and no thinking, and *samprajnata samadhi* is the state in which there are no thoughts, but thinking is perfect. This distinction has to be understood.

Your thoughts, in the first place, are not yours. You have gathered them. Just in a dark room, sometimes a beam of light comes from the roof and you see millions of dust particles floating in the beam. When I look into you, I see the same phenomenon: millions of dust particles. You call them thoughts. They are moving in you and out of you. From one head they enter another, and they go on. They have their own life.

A thought is a thing; it has its own existence. When a person dies, all his mad thoughts are released immediately and they start finding shelter somewhere or other. Immediately those who are around they enter. They are like germs: they have their own life. Even when you are alive, you go on dispersing your thoughts all around you. When you talk, then, of course, you throw your thoughts into others. But when you are silent, then also you are throwing thoughts all around. They are not yours, the first thing.

A man of positive reasoning will discard all thoughts that are not his own. They are not authentic; he has not found them through his own experience. He has accumulated from others, borrowed. They are dirty. They have been in many hands and heads. A man of thinking will not borrow. He would like to have a fresh thought of his own. And if you are positive, and if you look at the beauty, at the truth, at the goodness, at the flowers, if you become capable of seeing even in the darkest night that the morning is coming nearer, you will become capable of thinking.

Then you can create your own thoughts. And a thought that is created by you is really potential: it has a power of its own. These thoughts that you have borrowed are almost dead because they have been traveling — traveling for millions of years. Their origin is lost: they have lost all contact with their origin. They are just like dust floating all around. You catch them. Sometimes you even become aware of it, but because your awareness is such that it cannot see through things. . .

Sometimes you are sitting. Suddenly you become sad for no reason at all. You cannot find the reason. You look around, there is no reason; nothing there, nothing has happened. You are just the same and suddenly a sadness takes. A thought is passing; you are just in the way. It is an accident. A thought was passing like a cloud — a sad thought released by someone. It is an accident. You are in the grip. Sometimes a thought persists. You don't see why you go on thinking about it. It looks absurd; it seems to be of no use. But you cannot do anything. It goes on knocking at the gate. "Think me," it says. A thought is waiting at the door knocking. It says, "Give space. I would like to come in."

Each thought has its own life. It moves. And it has much power, and you are so impotent because you are so unaware, so you are moved by thoughts. Your whole life consists of such accidents. You meet people, and your whole life pattern changes. Something enters in you. Then you become possessed, and you forget where you were going. You change your direction; you follow this thought. And this is just an accident. You are like children.

Patanjali says this is not thinking. This is the state of absence of thinking; this is not thinking. You are a crowd. You have not a center within you which can think. When one moves in the discipline of *vitarka* — right reasoning, then one becomes by and by capable of thinking. Thinking is a capacity; thoughts are not. Thoughts can be learned from others; thinking, never. Thinking you have to learn yourself.

And this is the difference between the old Indian schools of learning and the modern universities: in the modern universities you are getting thoughts; in the ancient schools of learning, wisdom schools, they were teaching thinking, not thoughts.

Thinking is a quality of your inner being. What does thinking mean? It means to retain your consciousness, to remain alert and aware, to encounter a problem. A problem is there: you face it with your total awareness. And then arises an answer—a response. This is thinking. A question is posed; you have a ready-made answer. Before even you have thought about it, the answer comes in. Somebody says, "Is there God?" And he has not even said and you say, "Yes." You nod your wooden head; you say, "Yes, there is."

Is it your thought? Have you thought about the problem right now, or you carry a ready-made answer within your memory? Somebody gave it to you—your parents, your teachers, your society. Somebody has given it to you, and you carry it as a precious treasure, and this answer comes from that memory.

A man of thinking uses his consciousness each time there is a problem. Freshly, he uses his consciousness. He encounters the problem, and then arises a thought within him which is not part of memory. This is the difference. A man of thoughts is a man of memory; he has no thinking capacity. If you ask a question which is new, he will be at a loss. He cannot answer. If you ask a question which he knows the answer, he will immediately answer. This is the difference between a pundit and a man who knows; a man who can think.

Patanjali says *vitarka*—right reasoning, leads to reflection—*vichar*. Reflection—*vichar*, leads to bliss. This is the first glimpse, of course, and it is a glimpse. It will come and it will be lost. You cannot hold it for long. It was going to be just a glimpse, as if for a moment a lightning happened and you saw all darkness disappeared. But again the darkness is there—as if clouds disappeared and you saw the moon for a second —again clouds are there.

Or, on a sunny morning, near the Himalayas, for a moment you can have the glimpse of the Gourishankar —the highest peak. But then there is mist, and then there are clouds, and the peak is lost. This is *satori*. That's why never try to translate *satori* as *samadhi*. *Satori* is a glimpse. Much has to be done after it is attained. In fact, the real work starts after the first *satori*, first glimpse, because then you have tasted of the infinite. Now a real authentic search starts. Before it, it was just so-so, lukewarm, because you were not really confident, certain, what you are doing, where you are going, what is happening.

Before it, it was a faith, a trust. Before it a Master was needed to show you, to bring you back again and again. But after *satori* has happened, now it is no more a faith. It has become a knowing. Now the trust is not an effort. Now you trust because your own experience has shown you. After the first glimpse, the real search starts. Before it you are just going round and round. Right reasoning leads to right reflection, right reflection leads to a state of bliss, and this state of bliss leads to a sense of pure being.

A negative mind is always egoist. That is the impure state of being. You feel "I", but you feel "I" for wrong reasons. Just watch. Ego feeds on no. Whenever you say no, ego arises. Whenever you say yes, ego cannot arise because ego needs fight, ego needs challenge, ego needs to put itself against someone, something. It cannot exist alone; it needs duality. An egoist is always in search of fight—with someone, with something, with some situation. He is always trying to find something to say no —to win over, to be victorious.

Ego is violent, and no is the subtlest violence. When

you say no for ordinary things, even there ego arises. A small child says to the mother, "Can I go out to play?" and she says "No!" Nothing much was involved, but when the mother says "No!" she feels she is someone. You go to the railway station and you ask for a ticket and the clerk simply doesn't look at you. He goes on working even if there is no work. But he is saying, "No! Wait!" He feels he is someone, somebody. That's why, in offices everywhere, you will hear no. Yes is rare — very rare. An ordinary clerk can say no to anybody, whomsoever you are. He feels powerful.

No gives you a sense of power — remember this. Unless it is absolutely necessary, never say no. Even if it is absolutely necessary, say it in such an affirmative way that the ego doesn't arise. You can say. Even no can be said in such a way that it appears like yes. You can say yes in such a way that it looks like no. It depends on the tone; it depends on the attitude; it depends on the gesture.

Remember this: for seekers, it has to be remembered constantly that you have to live continuously in the aroma of yes. That is what a man of faith is: he says yes. Even when no was needed, he says yes. He doesn't see that there is any antagonism in life. He affirms. He says yes to his body, he says yes to his mind, he says yes to everybody, he says yes to the total existence. The ultimate flowering happens when you can say a categorical yes, with no conditions. Suddenly the ego falls; it cannot stand. It needs the props of no. The negative attitude creates ego. The positive attitude — the ego drops, and then the being is pure.

Sanskrit has two words for "I" — *ahankar* and *asmita*. It is difficult to translate. *Ahankar* is the wrong sense of "I" which comes from saying no. *Asmita* is the right sense of "I" which comes from saying yes. Both are "I". One is impure: no is the impurity. You negate, destroy. No is destructive, a very subtle destruction. Never use it. Drop it as much as you can. Whenever you are alert, don't use it. Try to find a roundabout way. Even if you have to say it, say it in such a way that it has the appearance of yes. By and by you will become attuned, and you will feel such a purity coming to you through yes.

Then *asmita: asmita* is egoless ego. No feeling of "I" against anybody. Just feeling oneself without putting against anybody. Just feeling your total loneliness, and the total loneliness, the purest of states. "I am"—when we say "I" is *ahankar;* "am" is *asmita,* just the feeling of am-ness with no "I" to it, just feeling the existence, the being. Yes is beautiful, no is ugly.

> *In* asamprajnata samadhi, *there is a cessation of all mental activity, and the mind only retains unmanifested impressions.*

*Samprajnata samadhi* is the first step. Right reasoning, right reflection, a state of bliss, a glimpse of bliss, and a feeling of am-ness—pure simple existence without any ego in it—this leads to *asamprajnata samadhi.* First is a purity; second is a disappearance because even the purest is impure because it is there. "I" is wrong; "am" is also wrong—better than "I", but a higher possibility is there when "am" also disappears—not only *ahankar,* but *asmita* also. You are impure; then you become pure. But if you start feeling that "I am pure", purity itself has become impurity. That too has to disappear.

Disappearance of the impurity is *samprajnata.* Disappearance of the purity also, is *asamprajnata.* There is a cessation of all mental activity. Thoughts disappear in the first state. In the second state, thinking also disappears. Thorns disappear in the first state. In the second state, flowers also disappear. When no disappears in the first state, yes remains. In the second state, yes also disappears because yes is also related to no. How can you retain yes without no? They are together; you cannot separate them. If no disappears, how can you say yes? Deep down yes is saying no to no. Negation of negation—but a subtle no exists. When you say yes, what you are doing? You are not saying no, but the no is inside. You are not bringing it out: it is unmanifested.

Your yes cannot mean anything if you have no "no" within you. What it will mean? It will be meaningless. Yes has meaning only because of no; no has meaning only because of yes. They are a duality. In *samprajnata samadhi*, no is dropped: all that is wrong is dropped. In *asamprajnata samadhi*, yes is dropped. All that is right, all that is good, that too is dropped. In *samprajnata samadhi* you drop the devil; in *asamprajnata samadhi* you drop the God also, because how the God can exist without the devil? They are two aspects of the same coin.

All activity ceases. Yes is also an activity, and activity is a tension. Something is going on, even beautiful but still something is going on. And after a period even the beautiful becomes ugly. After a period you are bored with flowers also. After a period, activity, even very subtle and pure, gives you a tension: it becomes an anxiety.

> In asamprajnata samadhi *there is a cessation of all activity, and the mind only retains unmanifested impressions.*

But still, it is not the goal — because what will happen to all your impressions that you have gathered in the past? Many, many lives you have lived, acted, reacted. You have done many things, undone many things. What will happen to it? Conscious mind has become pure; conscious mind has dropped even the activity of purity. But the unconscious is vast and there you carry all the seeds, the blueprints. They are within you.

The tree has disappeared; you have cut down the tree completely. But the seeds that have fallen, they are in the ground lying. They will sprout when their season comes. You will have another life; you will be born again. Of course, your quality will be different now, but you will be born again because those seeds are still not burned.

You have cut down that which was manifested. It is easy to cut down anything that is in manifestation; it is easy to cut all the trees. You can go into the garden and pull up all the whole lawn, the grass completely; you can kill everything. But within two weeks the grass will be coming up again because what you did is only with the manifested. The seeds which are lying in the soil you have not touched them yet. That has to be done in the third state.

*Asamprajnata samadhi* is still *sabeej* — with seeds. And there are methods how to burn those seeds, how to create fire — fire that Heraclitus talked about, how to create that fire and burn the unconscious seeds. When they also disappear, then the soil is absolutely pure; nothing can arise out of it. Then there is no birth, no death. Then the whole wheel stops for you; you have dropped out of the wheel. And dropping out of the society won't help unless you drop out of the wheel. Then you become a perfect drop-out.

A Buddha is a perfect drop-out; a Mahavira, a Patanjali, is a perfect drop-out. They have not dropped out of the establishment or the society. They have dropped out of the very wheel of life and death. But that happens only when all the seeds are burned. The final is *nirbeej samadhi* — seedless.

> In asamprajnata samadhi *there is a cessation of all mental activity, and the mind only retains unmanifested impressions.*

> Videhas *and* prakriti-layas *attain* asamprajnata samadhi *because they ceased to identify themselves with their bodies in their previous life. They take rebirth because seeds of desire remained.*

Even a Buddha is born. In his past life he attained to *asamprajnata samadhi*, but the seeds were there. He had

to come once more. Even a Mahavira is born — once —
the seeds bring him. But this is going to be the last life.
After *asamprajnata samadhi*, only one life is possible.
But then the quality of the life will be totally different
because this man will not be identified with the body.
And this man really has nothing to do because the
activity of the mind has ceased. Then what he will do?
For what this one life is needed? He has just to allow
those seeds to be manifested, and he will remain a witness. This is the fire.

One man came and spat on Buddha; he was angry.
Buddha wiped his face and asked, "What else you have
to say?" The man could not understand. He was really
angry — red-hot. He could not even understand what
Buddha is saying. And the whole thing was so absurd,
because Buddha didn't react. The man was at loss what
to do, what to say. He went away; the whole night he
couldn't sleep. How can you sleep when you insult
somebody and there is no reaction? Then your insult
comes back to yourself. You threw the arrow; it has not
been received. It comes back: it comes back to the
source finding no shelter. He insulted Buddha, but the
insult couldn't find a shelter there. So where it will go? It
comes to the original master.

The whole night he was feverish; he couldn't believe
what has happened. And then he started repenting, that
he was wrong — that he had not done good. The next
morning, early, he went and he asked for forgiveness.
Buddha said, "Don't be worried about it. I must have
done something wrong to you in the past. Now the
account is closed. And I am not going to react. Otherwise again and again. . . Finished! I have not reacted.
Because it was a seed somewhere, it has to be finished.
Now my account with you is closed."

In this life when a *videha* — one who has understood
that he is not the body, who has attained *asamprajnata
samadhi* — comes in the world just to finish accounts. . .
His whole life consists of finishing accounts; millions of

lives, many relationships, many involvements, commitments—everything has to be closed.

It happened: Buddha came to a village. The whole
village gathered; they were eager to listen him. It was a
rare opportunity. Even capitals were inviting continuously Buddha, and he was not coming. And he has
come to this small village out of the way—and without
any invitation, because the villagers never could gather
courage to go and ask him to come their village—just a
small village, few huts, and he has come without any
invitation. The whole village is afire with excitement,
and he is sitting under the tree and not speaking.

And they said, "For whom you are waiting now?
Everybody is here; the whole village is here. You start."
Buddha said, "But I have to wait because I have come
for someone who is not here. A promise has to be fulfilled, an account closed. I am waiting for that one."
Then came a girl, and then Buddha started. Then after
he talked, they asked, "Were you waiting for this girl?"

Because the girl belonged to the untouchables—to the
lowest caste, nobody could think of Buddha waiting for
her. He said, "Yes, I was waiting for her. When I was
coming she has met me on the road and she said, 'Wait,
because I am going for some work to the other town.
But I will come soon.' And in past lives somewhere I had
given her a promise that when I become enlightened I
will come and say whatsoever has happened to me.
That account has to be closed. That promise is hanging
on me, and if I can not fulfill it, I will have to come
again."

A *videha* or a *prakriti-laya*: both words are beautiful. *Videha* means bodiless. When you attain to *asamprajnata samadhi* the body is there, but you become
bodiless. You are no more the body. The body becomes
the abode; you are not identified.

So these two terms are beautiful. *Videha* means one
who knows that he is not the body—knows, remember
—not believes. And *prakriti-laya*, because one who

knows that he is not the body, he is no more the *prakriti*
— the nature.

Body belongs to the material. Once you are not
identified with the matter in you, you are not identified
with the matter without, outside. A man who attains
that he is no more the body, that he is no more the
manifested — the *prakriti* — his nature is dissolved. There
is no more world for him; he is not identified. He has
become a witness to it. Such a man is also born once at
least because he has to close many accounts, many
promises to be fulfilled, many karmas to be dropped.

It happened that Buddha's cousin, Devadatta, was
against him. He tried to kill him in many ways. When
Buddha was waiting under a tree meditating, he rolled
down a big rock from the hill. The rock was coming;
everybody ran away. Buddha remained there sitting
under the tree. It was dangerous, and the rock came just
touching him, brushing him. Ananda asked him, "Why
didn't you escape when we were all escaping? There was
time enough."

Buddha says, "For you there is time enough. My time
is over. And Devadatta has to do it. Some time back in
some life there was some karma. I must have given him
some pain, some anguish, some anxiety. It has to be
closed. If I escape, if I do anything, again a new line
starts."

A *videha*, a man who has attained to *asamprajnata*,
does not react. He simply watches, witnesses. And this
is the fire of witnessing which burns all the seeds in the
unconscious. And a moment comes when the soil is
absolutely pure. There is no seed waiting to sprout.
Then there is no need to come back. First the nature
dissolves, and then he dissolves himself into the universe.

Videhas *and* prakriti-layas *attain* asamprajnata
samadhi *because they ceased to identify
themselves with their bodies in their previous*

*life. They take rebirth because seeds of desire
remained.*

I am here to fulfill something; you are here to close my
account. You are here not accidentally. There are millions of people in the world. Why you are here, and not
somebody else? Something has to be closed.

*Others who attain* asamprajnata samadhi *attain
through faith, effort, recollection, concentration
and discrimination.*

So these are the two possibilities. If you have attained to
*asamprajnata samadhi* in your past life, in this life you
are born a Buddha—just a few seeds which have to be
fulfilled, which have to be dropped, burned—almost.
That's why I say you are born almost a Buddha. There is
no need for you to do anything; you have simply to
watch whatsoever happens.

Hence, Krishnamurti's continuous insistence that
there is no need to do anything. It is right for him; it is
not right for his listeners. For his listeners, there is much
to be done, and they will be misguided by this statement. He is speaking about himself. He was born an
*asamprajnata* Buddha. He was born a *videha*; he was
born a *prakriti-laya*.

He was taking a bath when he was just five years old
near Adyar, and one of the greatest Theosophists, Leadbeater, watched him. He was totally a different type of
child. If somebody was throwing mud on him, he will
not react. There were many children playing. If somebody will push him into the river, he will simply go.
Yes, he was not angry, he was not fighting. He has a
totally different quality—the quality of an *asamprajnata* Buddha.

Leadbeater called Annie Besant to watch this child.
He is no ordinary child, and the whole Theosophical
movement whirled around him. They hoped much that
he will become an *avatar*—that he will become the

perfect Master for this age. But the problem was deep.
They had chosen a right person, but they hoped wrong-
ly—because a man who is born an *asamprajnata* Buddha cannot even be active as an *avatar*. Because all
activity ceased. He can simply watch; he can be a
witness. You cannot make him very active. He can be
only a passivity. They had chosen the right person, but
still wrong.

And they hoped much. And then the whole movement whirled around Krishnamurti. And when he
dropped out of it, said, "I cannot do anything because
nothing is needed," the whole movement flopped because they hoped too much with this man, and then the
whole thing turned out completely different. But this
could have been prophesied.

Annie Besant, Leadbeater and others, they were
very, very beautiful persons, but not really aware of the
eastern methods. They have learned much from books,
scriptures, but they didn't know exactly the secret which
Patanjali is showing: that an *asamprajnata*, a *videha*, is
born, but he is not active. He is a passivity. Much can
happen through him, but that can happen only if somebody comes and surrenders to him. Because he is a
passivity, he cannot force you to do something. He is
available, but he cannot be aggressive.

His invitation is for everybody and all. It is an open
invitation, but he cannot send you an invitation in
particular, because he cannot be active. He is an open
door; if you like, you can pass. The last life is an absolute passivity, just witnessing. This is one way how
*asamprajnata* Buddhas are born from their past life.

But you can become an *asamprajnata* Buddha in this
life also. For them Patanjali says,

> Shraddha virya smriti samadhi prajna: *Others
> who attain* asamprajnata samadhi *attain through
> faith, effort, recollection, concentration and
> discrimination.*

It is almost impossible to translate it, so I will explain rather than translate, just to give you the feel, because words will misguide you.

*Shraddha* is not exactly faith. It is more like trust. Trust is very, very different from faith. Faith is something you are born in; trust is something you grow in. Hinduism is a faith; to be a Christian is a faith; to be a Mohammedan is a faith. But to be a disciple here with me is a trust. I cannot claim faith — remember. Jesus also could not claim faith because faith is something you are born in. Jews were faithful; they had faith. And, in fact, that is why they destroyed Jesus: because they thought that he was bringing them out of their faith, destroying their faith.

He was asking for trust. Trust is a personal intimacy; it is not a social phenomenon. You attain to it through your own response. Nobody can be born in trust; in faith, okay. Faith is dead trust; trust is alive faith. So try to understand the distinction.

*Shraddha* — trust — one has to grow in. And it is always personal. The first disciples of Jesus attained to trust. They were Jews, born Jews. They moved out of their faith. It is a rebellion. Faith is a superstition; trust is a rebellion. Trust first leads you away from your faith. It has to be so, because if you are living in a dead graveyard, then you have to be led out of it first. Only then you can be introduced to life again. Jesus was trying to bring people towards *shraddha*, trust. It will always look as if he is destroying their faith.

Now when a Christian comes to me, the same situation is again repeated. Christianity is a faith, just as Judaism was a faith in Jesus' time. When a Christian comes to me, again I have to bring him out of his faith to help him to grow towards trust. Religions are faith, and to be religious is to be in trust. And to be religious doesn't mean to be Christian, Hindu, or Mohammedan, because trust has no name; it is not labeled. It is like

love. Is love Christian, Hindu, Mohammedan? Marriage is Christian, Hindu, Mohammedan. Love? Love
knows no caste, no distinctions. Love knows no Hindus, no Christians.

Marriage is like faith; love is like trust. You have to
grow into it. It is an adventure. Faith is not an adventure. You are born into it; it is convenient. It is better if
you are seeking comfort and convenience, it is better to
remain in faith. Be a Hindu, a Christian; follow the
rules. But it will remain a dead thing unless you respond
from your heart, unless *you* enter religion on your own
responsibility, not that you were born a Christian. How
can you be a born Christian?

With birth how religion is associated? Birth cannot
give you religion; it can give you a society, a creed, a
sect; it can give you a superstition. The word "superstition" is very, very meaningful. It means "unnecessary
faith". The word "super" means unnecessary, superfluous—faith which has become unnecessary, faith
which has become dead; sometimes it may have been
alive. Religion has to be born again and again.

Remember, you are not born in a religion, religion
has to be born in you. Then it is trust. Again and again.
You cannot give your children your religion. They will
have to seek and find their own. Everybody has to seek
and find his own. It is adventure—the greatest adventure. You move into the unknown. *Shraddha*, Patanjali
says, is the first thing, if you want to attain *asamprajnata samadhi*. For *samaprajnata samadhi*, reasoning,
right reasoning. See the distinction? For *samprajnata
samadhi*, right reasoning, right thinking are the base;
for *asamprajnata samadhi*, right trust—not reasoning.

No reasoning—a love. And love is blind. It looks
blind to the reasoning because it is a jump into the dark.
The reason asks, "Where are you going? Remain in the
known territory. And what is the use to move to a new
phenomenon? Why not remain in the old fold? It is

convenient, comfortable, and whatsoever you need, it can supply." But everybody has to find his own temple. Only then it is alive.

You are here with me. This is a trust. When I am no more here, your children may be with me. That will be faith. Trust happens only with an alive Master; faith, with dead Masters which are no more there. The first disciples have the religion. The second, third generation by and by loses the religion, it becomes a sect. Then you simply follow because you are born into it. It is a duty, not a love. It is a social code. It helps, but it is nothing deep in you. It brings nothing to you; it is not a happening. It is not a depth unfolding in you. It is just a surface, a face. Just go and see in the church. The Sunday people, they go; they even pray. But they are waiting when this is finished.

A small child was sitting in a church. For the first time he had come, just four years of age. The mother asked him, "How you liked it?" He said, "Music is good, but the commercial is too long." It is commercial when you have no trust. *Shraddha* is right trust; faith is wrong trust. Don't take religion from somebody else. You cannot borrow it; it is a deception. You are getting it without paying for it, and everything has to be paid. And it is not cheap to attain to *asamprajnata samadhi*. You have to pay the full cost, and the full cost is your total being.

To be a Christian is just a label; to be religious is not a label. Your whole being is involved. It is a commitment. People come to me and they say, "We love you. Whatsoever you say is good. But we don't want to take sannyas because we don't want to be committed." But unless you are committed, involved, you cannot grow, because then there is no relationship. Between you and me then there are words, not a relationship. Then I may be a teacher, but I am not a Master to you. Then you may be a student, but not a disciple.

*Shraddha,* trust, is the first door; second is *virya.* That too is difficult. It is translated as effort. No, effort is simply a part of it. The word *virya* means many things, but deep down it means bio-energy. One of the meanings of *virya* is semen, the sexual potency. If you really want to translate it exactly, *virya* is bio-energy, your total energy phenomenon—you as energy. Of course, this energy can be brought only through effort; hence, one of the meanings is "effort".

But that is poor—not so rich as the word *virya. Virya* means that your total energy has to be brought into it. Only mind won't do. You can say yes from the mind, that will not be enough. Your totality, without holding anything back: that is the meaning of *virya.* And that is possible only when there is trust. Otherwise you will hold something, just to be secure, safe, because, "This man may be leading somewhere wrong, so we can step back any moment. In a moment we can say 'Enough is enough; now no more.' "

You hold back a part of you just to be watchful, where this man is leading. People come to me and they say, "We are watching. Let us first watch what is happening." They are very clever—clever fools—because these things cannot be watched from the outside. What is happening is an inner phenomenon. Even you cannot see to whom it is happening many times. Many times only I can see what is happening. You become aware only later on, what has happened.

Others cannot watch. From the outside there is no possibility to watch it. How can you watch from the outside? Gestures you can see; people doing meditation you can see. But what is happening inside, that is meditation. What they are doing outside is just creating a situation.

It happened: there was a very great Sufi Master, Jalaludin. He had a small school of rare pupils, rare, because he was a very choosy one. He would not allow anybody unless he had chosen. For very few he worked, but people passing sometimes would come to see what was happening there. Once a group of people came, professors. They are always very alert people, very clever, and they looked. In the Master's house, just in the compound, a group of fifty people were sitting, and they were doing mad gestures—somebody laughing, somebody crying, somebody jumping. The professors watched.

They said, "What is going on? This man is leading them toward madness. They are already mad, and they are fools—because once you become mad it will be difficult to come back. And this is nonsense; we have never heard. People when they meditate, they sit silently."

And there was much discussion between them. A group of them said, "Because we don't know what is happening, it is not good to take any judgment." Then there was a third group among them who said, "Whatsoever it is, it is worth enjoying. We would like to watch. It is beautiful. Why can't we enjoy it? Why be bothered what they are doing? But just to watch them is a beautiful thing."

Then after a few months, again, the same group came to the school to watch. Now what was happening? Now everybody was silent. The fifty persons were there, the Master was there—they were sitting silently, so silently, as if there was no one, like statues. Again there was discussion. There was a group who said, "Now they are useless. What to see? Nothing! The first time we had come it was beautiful. We had enjoyed it. But now they are just boring." The other group said, "But now we think they are meditating. The first time they were simply mad. This is the right thing to do; this is how meditation is done. It is written in the scriptures, described in this way."

But there was still a third group who said, "We don't

know anything about meditation. How can we judge?"

Then, again, after a few months, the group came. Now there was nobody. Only the Master was sitting, smiling. All the disciples had disappeared. So they asked, "What is happening? The first time we came there was a mad crowd, and we thought this is useless, you are driving people crazy. The next time we came it was very good. People were meditating. Where have they all gone?"

The Master said, "The work done, the disciples have disappeared. And I am smiling happy because the thing happened. And you are the fools, I know! I have also been watching — not only you. I know what discussions were going on, and what you were thinking the first time and the second time." Said Jalaludin, "The effort that you have taken to come here for three times would have been enough for you to become meditators. And the discussion that you have been in, that much energy was enough to make you silent. And in the same period, those disciples have disappeared, and you are standing at the same place. Come in! Don't watch from the outside." They said, "Yes! That is why we are coming again and again, to watch what is happening. When we are certain, then. . . Otherwise we don't want to be committed."

Clever people never want to be committed, but is there any life without commitment? But clever people think commitment is a bondage. But is there any freedom without bondage? First you have to move in a relationship, only then you can go beyond it. First you have to move in a deep commitment, depth to depth, heart to heart, and only then you can transcend it. There is no other way. If you just move out and watch, you can never enter into the shrine — the shrine is commitment. And then there can be no relationship.

A Master and disciple is a love relationship, the highest love that is possible. Unless the relationship is there, you cannot grow. Says Patanjali, "The first is trust — *shraddha* — and second is energy — effort." Your whole energy has to be brought in; part won't do. It may even be destructive if you come only partially in and remain partially out, because that will become a rift within you. It will create a tension within you; it will become an anxiety rather than bliss.

Bliss is where you are in your totality; anxiety is where you are only in part, because then you are divided and there is a tension, and the two parts going separate ways. Then you are in a difficulty.

> "*Others who attain* asamprajnata samadhi *attain through faith, trust, effort, energy, recollection.*"

This word recollection is *smriti*: it is remembrance — what Gurdjieff calls self-remembering. That is *smriti*.

You don't remember yourself. You may remember millions of things, but you go on continuously forgetting yourself, that you are. Gurdjieff had a technique. He got it from Patanjali. And, in fact, all techniques come from Patanjali. He is the past Master of techniques. *Smriti*, remembrance — self-remembering — whatsoever you do. You are walking: remember deep down that "I am walking, I am." Don't be lost in walking. Walking is there — the movement, the activity — and the inner center is there, just aware, watching, witnessing.

You need not repeat it in the mind, "I am walking." If you repeat, that is not remembrance. You have to be non-verbally aware that "I am walking, I am eating, I am talking, I am listening." Whatsoever you do, the "I" inside should not be forgotten; it should remain. It is not self-consciousness. It is consciousness of the self. Self-consciousness is ego; consciousness of the self is *asmita* — purity, just being aware that "I am".

Ordinarily, your consciousness is arrowed towards the object. You look at me: your whole consciousness is moving towards me like an arrow. But you are arrowed towards me. Self-remembering means you must have a double-arrowed arrow, one side of it showing to me, another side showing to you. A double-arrowed arrow is *smriti* — self-remembrance.

Very difficult, because it is easy to remember the object and forget yourself. The opposite is also easy — to remember yourself and forget the object. Both are easy; that's why those who are in the market, in the world, and those who are in the monastery, out of the world, are the same. Both are single-arrowed. In the market they are looking at the things, objects. In the monastery they are looking at themselves.

*Smriti* is neither in the market nor in the monastery. *Smriti* is a phenomenon of self-remembering, when subject and object both are together in consciousness. That is the most difficult thing in the world. Even if you can attain for a single moment, a split moment, you will have the glimpse of *satori* immediately. Immediately you have moved out of the body, somewhere else.

Try it. But, remember, if you don't have trust it will become a tension. These are the problems involved. It will become such a tension you can go mad, because it is a very tense state. That's why it is difficult to remember both — the object and the subject, the outer and the inner. To remember both is very, very arduous. If there is trust, that trust will bring the tension down because trust is love. It will soothe you; it will be a soothing force around you. Otherwise the tension can become so much, you will not be able to sleep. You will not be able to be at peace any moment because it will be a constant problem. And you will be just in anxiety continuously.

That's why we can do one: that's easy. Go to the monastery, close your eyes, remember yourself, forget the world. But what you are doing? You have simply reversed the whole process, nothing else. No change. Or, forget these monasteries and these temples and these

Masters, and be in the world, enjoy the world. That too is easy. The difficult thing is to be conscious of the both. And when you are conscious of the both and the energy is simultaneously aware, arrowed in the diametrically opposite dimensions, there is a transcendence. You simply become the third: you become the witness of both. And when the third enters, first you try to see the object and yourself. But if you try to see both, by and by, by and by, you feel something is happening within you — because you are becoming a third: you are between the two, the object and the subject. You are neither the object nor the subject now.

*Attain through faith, effort, recollection,*
*concentration and discrimination.*

*Shraddha*, trust, *virya*, total commitment, total effort, total energy has to be brought in; all your potentiality has to be brought in. If you are really a seeker after truth, you cannot seek anything else. It is a complete involvement. You cannot make it a part-time job and that, "Sometimes in the morning I meditate and then I go." No, meditation has to become your twenty-four-hours continuity for you. Whatsoever you do, meditation has to be there in the background continuously. Energy will be needed: your whole energy will be needed.

And now, few things. If your whole energy is needed, sex disappears automatically because you don't have energy to waste. *Brahmacharya* for Patanjali is not a discipline, it is a consequence. You put your total energy so you don't have any energy. . .and it happens in ordinary life also. You can see a great painter: he forgets women completely. When he is painting there is no sex in his mind, because the whole energy is moving. You don't have any extra energy.

A great poet, a great singer, a dancer who is moving totally in his commitment, automatically becomes celibate. He has no discipline for it. Sex is superfluous energy; sex is a safety valve. When you have too much in you and you cannot do anything with it, the nature has made a safety valve; you can throw it out. You can release it, otherwise you will go mad or burst — explode. And if you try to suppress it, then too you will go mad, because suppressing it won't help. It needs a transformation, and that transformation comes from total commitment. A warrior, if he is really a warrior — an impeccable warrior, will be beyond sex. His whole energy is moving.

It is reported, a very, very beautiful story: a great philosopher, thinker, his name was Vachaspati. . . He was so much involved in his studies that when his father asked him that, "Now I am getting old, and I don't know when I will die — any moment — and you are my only son, and I would like you to be married." He was so much involved in his studies that he said, "Okay." He didn't hear what he was saying. So he got married. He got married, but he completely forgot that he has a wife, he was so involved.

And this can happen only in India; this cannot happen anywhere else: the wife loved him so much that she didn't want to disturb. So it is said twelve years passed. She will serve him like a shadow, take every care, but not to disturb, not to say that, "I am here, and what you are doing?" Continuously he was writing a commentary — one of the greatest ever written. He was writing a commentary on Badarayan's *Brahm-Sutras* and he was so involved, so totally, that he not only forgot about his wife: he was not even aware who brings the food, who takes the plates back, who comes in the evening and lights the lamp, who prepares his bed.

Twelve years passed, and the night came when his commentary was complete. Just the last word he was to write, and he had taken a vow, and when the commentary is complete he will become a sannyasin. Then he will not be concerned with the mind, and everything is finished. This is his only karma that has to be fulfilled.

That night he was a little relaxed, because the last sentence he wrote nearabout twelve, and for the first time he became aware of the surroundings. The lamp was burning low and needed more oil. A beautiful hand was pouring oil into it. He looked back who is there. He couldn't recognize the face; he said, "Who are you and what are you doing here?" The wife said, "Now that you have asked, I must say that twelve years back you had brought me as your wife, but you were so much involved, so much committed to your work, I didn't like to interrupt or disturb you."

Vachaspati started weeping, his tears started flowing. The wife asked, "What is the matter?" He said, "This is very complex. Now I am at a loss, because the commentary is complete and I am a sannyasin. I cannot be a householder; I cannot be your husband. The commentary is complete, and I had taken a vow and now there is no time for me, I am going to leave immediately. Why didn't you tell me before? I could have loved you. And what can I do for your services, your love, your devotion?"

So he called his commentary on *Brahm-Sutras*, *Bhamati*. *Bhamati* was the name of his wife. The name is absurd, because to call Badarayan's *Brahm-Sutras* and the commentary, *Bhamati*, it has no relationship. But he said, "Now nothing else I can do. The last thing is to write the name of the book, so I will call it *Bhamati* so that it is always remembered."

He left the house. The wife was weeping, crying, but not in pain but in absolute bliss. She said, "That's enough. This gesture, this love in your eyes, is enough. I have got enough; don't feel guilty. Go! And forget me completely. I would not like to be a burden on your mind. No need to remember me."

It is possible, if you are involved totally, sex disappears because sex is a safety valve. When you have energy unused, then sex becomes a haunting thing around you. When total energy is used, sex disappears. And that is the state of *brahmacharya*, of *virya*, of all your potential energy flowering.

*Effort, recollection, concentration and discrimination:*

*Shraddha* — trust; *virya* — your total bio-energy, your total commitment and effort; *smriti* — self-remembrance; and *samadhi*. *Samadhi* word means a state of mind where no problem exists. It comes from the word *samadhan* — a state of mind when you feel absolutely okay, no problem, no question, a non-questioning, non-problematic state of mind. It is not concentration. Concentration is just a quality that comes to the mind who is without problems. That is the difficulty to translate.

Concentration is part — it happens. Look at a child who is absorbed in his play; he has a concentration without any effort. He is not concentrating on his play. Concentration is a byproduct. He is so absorbed in the play that the concentration happens. If you concentrate knowingly on something, then there is effort, then there is tension, then you will be tired.

*Samadhi* happens automatically, spontaneously, if you are absorbed. If you are listening to me, it is a *samadhi*. If you listen to me totally, there is no need for any other meditation. It becomes a concentration. It is not that you concentrate — if you listen lovingly, concentration follows.

In *asamprajnata samadhi*, when trust is complete, when effort is total, when remembrance is deep, *samadhi* happens. Whatsoever you do, you do with total concentration — without any effort to do the concentration. And if concentration needs effort, it is ugly. It will be like a disease on you; you will be destroyed by it. Concentration should be a consequence. You love a person, and just being with him, you are concentrated. Remember never to concentrate on anything. Rather, listen deeply, listen totally, and you will have a concentration coming by itself.

And discrimination — *prajna*. *Prajna* is not discrimination; discrimination is again a part of *prajna*. *Prajna* means in fact wisdom — a knowing awareness. Buddha has said that when the flame of meditation burns high, the light that surrounds that flame is *prajna*. *Samadhi* inside, and then all around you a light, an aura, follows you. In your every act you are wise; not that you are trying to be wise, it simply happens because you are so totally aware. Whatsoever you do it happens to be wise — not that you are continuously thinking to do the right thing.

A man who is continuously thinking to do the right thing, he will not be able to do anything — even the wrong he will not be able to do, because this will become such a tension on his mind. And what is right and what is wrong? How you can decide? A man of wisdom, a man of understanding, does not choose. He simply feels. He simply throws his awareness everywhere, and in that light he moves. Wherever he moves is right.

Right does not belong to things; it belongs to you — the one who is moving. It is not that Buddha did right things — no! Whatsoever he did was right. Discrimination is a poor word. A man of understanding has discrimination. He doesn't think about it; just it is easy for him. If you want to get out of this room, you simply move out of the door. You don't grope. You don't first go to the wall and try to find the way. You simply go out. You don't even think that this is the door.

But when a blind man has to go out, he asks, "Where is the door?" And then too he tries to find it. He will knock many places with his cane, he will grope, and continuously in the mind he will think, "Is it the door or the wall? Am I going right or wrong?" And when he comes to the door, he thinks, "Yes, now this is the door."

All this happens because he is blind. You have to

discriminate because you are blind; you have to think because you are blind; you have to believe in right and wrong because you are blind; you have to be in discipline and morality because you are blind. When understanding flowers, when the flame is there, you simply see and everything is clear. When you have an inner clarity, everything is clear; you become perceptive. Whatsoever you do is simply right. Not that it is right so you do it; you do it with understanding, and it is right.

*Shraddha, virya, smriti, samadhi, prajna.* Others who attain *asamprajnata samadhi* attain through trust, infinite energy, effort, total self-remembrance, a non-questioning mind and a flame of understanding.

# Attraction To The Difficult

The first question:

*What you have been saying about Heraclitus,
Christ and Zen seems like kindergarten teachings
compared to Patanjali. Heraclitus, Christ and
Zen make the final step seem close; Patanjali
makes even the first step seem almost
impossible. It seems like us westerners have
hardly begun to realize the amount of work that
has to be done.*

SAYS LAO TZU, "IF TAO IS NOT
laughed at, it will not be Tao." And
I would like to say to you: If you
will not misunderstand me, you will
not be you. You are bound to
misunderstand. You have not understood
what I had been saying about Heraclitus,
Christ and Zen, and if you cannot
understand Heraclitus, Zen and Jesus, you
will not be able to understand Patanjali
either.

The first rule of understanding is not to compare. How
can you compare? What do you know about the innermost state of Heraclitus or Basho or Buddha, Jesus or
Patanjali? Who are you to compare?—because comparison is a judgment. Who are you to judge? But the
mind wants to judge because in judgment the mind feels

superior. You become the judge; your ego feels very, very good. You feed the ego. Through judgment and comparison you think that you know.

They are different types of flowers — incomparable. How can you compare a rose with a lotus? Is there any possibility to compare? There is no possibility because both are different worlds. How can you compare moon with the sun? There is no possibility. They are different dimensions. Heraclitus is a wild flower; Patanjali is in a cultivated garden. Patanjali will be nearer your intellect, Heraclitus nearer your heart. But as you go deeper, the differences are lost. When you yourself start flowering, then a new understanding dawns upon you — the understanding that flowers differ in their color, they differ in their smell, they differ in their shape, form and name.

But in flowering they don't differ. The flowering, the phenomenon that they have flowered, is the same. Heraclitus is, of course, different; has to be. Every individual is unique; Patanjali is different. You cannot put them into one category. There exist no pigeonholes where you can force them, categorize them. But if you also flower, then you will come to understand that flowering is the same whether the flower is lotus or rose — makes no difference. The innermost phenomenon of energy coming to a celebration is the same.

They talk differently; they have different patterns of mind. Patanjali is a scientific thinker. He is a grammarian, a linguist. Heraclitus is a wild poet. He does not bother about grammar and language and the form. And when you say that listening to Patanjali, you feel that Heraclitus and Basho and Zen they appear childish, kindergarten teachings, you are not saying anything about Patanjali or Heraclitus, you are saying something about you. You are saying that you are a mind-oriented person.

Patanjali you can understand; Heraclitus simply eludes you. Patanjali is more solid. You can have a grip.

Heraclitus is a cloud; you cannot have any grip on him. Patanjali, you can make tail and head out of him; he seems rational. What you will do with a Heraclitus, with a Basho? No, simply they are so irrational. Thinking about them, your mind becomes absolutely impotent. When you say such things, comparisons, judgments, you say something about you—that who you are.

Patanjali can be understood; there is no trouble about it. He is absolutely rational, can be followed, no problem about it. All his techniques can be done because he gives you the how, and how is always easy to understand. What to do? How to do? He gives you the techniques.

Ask Basho or Heraclitus what to do, and they simply say there is nothing to be done. Then you are at a loss. If something is to be done you can do it, but if nothing is to be done you are at a loss. Still, you will go on asking again and again, "What to do? How to do? How to achieve this you are talking about?"

They talk about the ultimate without talking about the way that leads to it. Patanjali talks about the way, never talking about the goal. Patanjali is concerned with the means, Heraclitus with the end. The end is mysterious. It is a poetry; it is not a mathematical solution. It is a mystery. But the path is a scientific thing, the technique, the know-how; it appeals you. But this shows something about you, not about Heraclitus or Patanjali. You are a mind-oriented person, a head-oriented person. Try to see this. Don't compare Patanjali and Heraclitus. Simply try to see the thing—that it shows something about you. And if it shows something about you, you can do something.

Don't think that you know what Patanjali is and what Heraclitus is. You can't even understand an ordinary flower in the garden, and they are the ultimate flowering in existence. Unless you flower in the same way, you will not be able to understand. But you can compare, you can judge, and through judgment you will miss the whole point.

So the first rule of understanding is never to judge. Never judge and never compare Buddha, Mahavira, Mohammed, Christ, Krishna; never compare! They exist in a dimension beyond comparison, and whatsoever you know about them is really nothing — just fragments. You cannot have the total comprehension. They are so beyond. In fact, you simply see their reflection in the water of your mind.

You have not seen the moon; you have seen the moon in the lake. You have not seen the reality; you have simply seen a mirror reflection, and the reflection depends on the mirror. If the mirror is defective, the reflection is different. Your mind is your mirror.

When you say that Patanjali seems to be very great, and teaching very great, you are simply saying that you couldn't understand Heraclitus at all. And if you cannot understand, that simply shows that he is very very beyond you than Patanjali; he is far beyond than Patanjali. At least you can understand this much — that Patanjali seems to be difficult. Now follow me closely. If something is difficult, you can tackle with. Howsoever difficult, you can tackle! More hard effort is needed, but that can be done.

Heraclitus is not easy; he is simply impossible. Patanjali is difficult. Difficult you can understand, you can do something, you can bring your will to it, your effort, your whole energy to it, and you can do something, and it can be solved. Difficult can be made easy, more subtle methods can be found. But what you will do with the impossible? It cannot be made easy. But you can deceive yourself. You can say there is nothing in it, it is a kindergarten teaching, and you are such a grown-up, it is not for you; it is for children, not for you.

This is a trick of the mind to avoid the impossible, because you know you will not be able to tackle it. So the only easiest course is simply to say, "It is not for me;

it is below me — a kindergarten teaching," and you are a grown-up mature person. You need a university; you don't need a kindergarten school. Patanjali suits you, looks very difficult, can be solved. The impossible cannot be solved.

If you want to understand Heraclitus, there is no way except you drop your mind completely. If you want to understand Patanjali, there is a way gradually. He gives you steps what to do; but remember, finally, eventually, he will also say to you, "Drop the mind." What Heraclitus says in the beginning, he will say in the end, but on the path, the whole way, you can be fooled. In the end he is going to say the same thing, but still he will be understandable because he makes grades, and the jump doesn't look like a jump when you have steps.

Just this is the situation: Heraclitus brings you to an abyss and says, "Jump!" You look down; your mind simply cannot comprehend what he is saying. It looks suicidal. There are no steps. And you ask, "How?" He says, "There is no 'how?', you simply jump. What is the 'how'?" Because there are no steps, so "how" cannot be explained. You simply jump, and he says, "If you are ready I can push you, but there are no methods." Is there any method to take a jump? Because jump is sudden. Methods exist when a thing, a process, is gradual. Finding it impossible, you turn about. But to console yourself that you are not such a weakling, you say, "This is for children. It is not difficult enough." It is not for you.

Patanjali brings you to the same abyss, but he has made steps. He says one step at a time. It appeals! You can understand! The mathematics is simple; take one step, then another. There is no jump. But, remember, sooner or later he will bring you to the point from where you have to jump. Steps he has created, but they don't lead to the bottom — just in the middle, and the bottom is so far away, you can exactly say it is a bottomless abyss.

So how many steps you make makes no difference. The abyss remains the same. He will lead you ninety-nine steps, and you are very happy—as if you have covered the abyss, and now the bottom has come nearer. No, the bottom remains as far away as before. These ninety-nine steps are just to befool your mind, just to give you a "how", a technique. Then at the hundredth step, he says, "Now jump!" And the abyss remains the same, the span the same.

No difference because the abyss is infinite, God is infinite. How can you meet him gradually? But these ninety-nine steps will befool you. Patanjali is more clever. Heraclitus is innocent: he simply says you, "This is the thing: the abyss is here. Jump!" He does not persuade you; he does not seduce you. He simply says, "This is the fact. If you want to jump, jump; if you don't want to jump, go away."

And he knows that to make steps is useless because finally one has to take the jump. But I think it will be good for you to follow Patanjali because, by and by, he seduces you. One step you can take at least, then the second becomes easier, then the third. And when you have taken ninety-nine steps, to go back will be difficult, because then it will look absolutely against your ego to go back: because then the whole world will laugh, and you had become such a great sage, and you are coming back to the world? And you were such a *maha-yogi*—a great yogi, and why you are coming back? Now you are caught, and you cannot go back.

Heraclitus is simple, innocent. His teaching is not of a kindergarten school, but he is a child—that's right—innocent like a child, wise also like a child. Patanjali is cunning, clever, but Patanjali will suit you because you need somebody who can lead you in a cunning way to a point from where you cannot go back. It becomes simply impossible.

Gurdjieff used to say that there are two types of Masters: one innocent and simple; another sly, cunning.

He himself said, "I belong to the second category." Patanjali is the source of all sly Masters. They lead you to the rose garden, and then, suddenly, the abyss. And you are caught in such a grip of your own making, that you cannot go back. You meditated, you renounced the world, renounced wife and children. For years you were doing postures, meditating, and you created such an aura around you that people worshipped you. Millions of people looked at you as a god, and now comes the abyss. Now just to save you have to jump: just to save your prestige. Where to go? Now you cannot go.

Buddha is simple; Patanjali is sly. All science is cunningness. This has to be understood, and I am not saying it in any derogatory sense, remember; I am not condemning. All science is cunningness!

It is said that one follower of Lao Tzu — an old man, a farmer — was drawing water from a well, and instead of using bullocks or horses, he himself — an old man — and his son, they were working like bullocks and carrying the water out of the well, perspiring, the old man, breathing hard. It was difficult.

A follower of Confucius was passing. He said to this old man, that "Have you not heard? This is very primitive. Why are you wasting your breath? Now bullocks can be used, horses can be used. Have you not heard that in the town, in the cities, how nobody is working like this that you are working? It is very primitive. Science has progressed fast."

The old man said, "Wait, and don't talk so loudly. When my son is gone, then I will reply." When the son was gone to do some work, he said, "Now you are a dangerous person. If my son ever hears about this, immediately he will say, 'Okay! Then I don't want to pull this. I can't do this work of a bullock. A bullock is needed.' "

The disciple of Confucius says, "What is wrong in that?" The old man said, "Everything is wrong in it because it is cunningness. It is deceiving the bullock; it is deceiving the horse. And one thing leads to another. And if this boy who is young and not wise, if he once knows that you can be cunning with animals, he will wonder why cannot you be cunning with man. Once he knows that through cunningness you can exploit, then I don't know where he will stop. You please go from here, and never come back again to this road. And don't bring such cunning things to this village. We are happy."

Lao Tzu is against science. He says science is cunningness. It is deceiving nature, exploiting nature — through cunning ways, forcing nature. And the more a man becomes scientific, the more cunning; has to be so. An innocent man cannot be scientific, difficult. But man has become cunning and clever. And Patanjali, knowing well that to be scientific is a cunningness, also knows that man can only be brought back to nature through a new device, a new cunningness.

Yoga is science of the inner being. Because you are not innocent, you have to be brought through a cunning way. If you are innocent, no means are needed, no methods are needed. A simple understanding, a childlike understanding, and you will be transformed. But you are not. That's why you feel that Patanjali seems to be very great. It is because of your head-oriented mind and your cunningness.

Second thing to remember: he appears difficult. And you think Heraclitus is simple? He appears difficult, that too becomes an appeal for the ego. The ego always wants to do something which is difficult, because against the difficult you feel you are someone. If something is very simple, how the ego can feed out of it?

People come to me and they say, "Sometimes you teach that just by sitting and doing nothing it can happen. How can it be so simple? How can it be so easy?" Says Chuang Tzu, "Easy is right," but these people say, "No! How can it be so easy? It must be difficult — very, very difficult, arduous."

You want to do difficult things because when you are

fighting against a difficulty, against the current, you feel you are someone — a conqueror. If something is simple, something is so easy that even a child can do it, then where your ego will stand? You ask for hurdles, you ask for difficulties, and if there are not difficulties you create, so that you can fight, so that you can fly against a strong wind and you can feel that, "I am someone — a conqueror!"

But don't be so smart. You know the phrase "smart aleck"? You may not know from where it comes — it comes from Alexander. The "aleck" word comes from Alexander, a short form. "Don't be a smart Alexander." Be simple: don't try to be a conqueror, because that is foolish. Don't try to be a somebody.

But Patanjali appealed; Patanjali appealed to the Indian ego very much, so India created the most subtle egoists in the world. You cannot find more subtle egoists anywhere in the world as you can find in India. It is almost impossible to find a simple yogi. Yogi cannot be simple, because he is doing so many *asanas*, so many *mudras*, and he is working so hard, how can he be simple? He thinks himself to be at the top — a conqueror. The whole world has to bow down to him; he is the cream — the very salt of life.

You go and watch yogis: you will find them very, very refined egos. Their inner shrine is still empty; the divine has not come in. That shrine is still a throne for their own egos. They may have become very subtle; they may have become so subtle that they may appear to be very humble, but in their humbleness also, if you watch, you will find the ego.

They are aware that they are humble, that's the difficulty. A really humble person is not aware that he is humble. A really humble person is simply humble, not aware, and a real humble person never claims that "I am humble," because all claims are of the ego. Humility cannot be claimed; humbleness is not a claim, it is a state of being. And all claims fulfill the ego. Why this happened? Why India became a very subtle-egoist country? And when there is ego, you become blind.

Now ask Indian yogis: they are condemning the whole world. West, they say it is materialist; only India is spiritual. The whole world is materialist, as if there is a monopoly. And they are so blind, they cannot see the fact that exactly opposite is the case.

The more I have been watching Indian and the western mind, I feel the western mind is less materialist than the Indian. The Indian mind is more materialist, clings to things more, cannot share, is miserly. The western mind can share, is less miserly. Because the West has created so much materialist affluence does not mean that the West is materialist, and because India is poor does not mean that you are spiritualists.

If poverty is spirituality, then impotence would be *brahmacharya*. No, poverty is not spirituality; neither affluence is materialism. Materialism doesn't belong to the things, it belongs to the attitude. Neither spirituality belongs to poverty, it belongs to the inner, non-attached, sharing. You cannot find in India anybody sharing anything. Nobody can share; everybody hoards. And because they are such hoarders, they are poor. Because few people hoard too much, then many people become poor.

The West has been sharing. That's why the whole society rises from poverty to affluence. In India, few people become so rich, you cannot find so rich people anywhere else — but few — and the whole society drags itself into poverty, and the gap is vast. You cannot find such a gap anywhere. The gap between a Birla and a beggar is vast. Such a gap cannot exist anywhere, is not in existence anywhere. Rich people are in the West, poor people are in the West, but the gap is not so vast. Here the gap is simply infinite. You cannot imagine such a gap. How can it be fulfilled? It cannot be fulfilled because the people are materialist. Otherwise how this gap? Why this gap? Can't you share? Impossible! But the ego says that the whole world, the whole world, is materialist.

This has come because people were attracted to Patanjali and to people who were giving difficult methods. Nothing is wrong with Patanjali, but Indian ego found a beautiful, subtle outlet to be egoist.

The same is happening to you. Patanjali appeals you; he is difficult. Heraclitus is "kindergarten" because he is so simple. Simplicity never appeals the ego. But, remember, if simplicity can become an appeal, the path is not long. If difficulty becomes the appeal, then the path is going to be very long because, from the very beginning, rather than dropping the ego, you have started accumulating it.

I am speaking on Patanjali not to make you more egoist. Look and watch. I am always afraid of talking about Patanjali; I am never afraid about talking Heraclitus, Basho, Buddha. I am afraid because of you. Patanjali is beautiful, but you can be attracted for wrong reasons, and this will be a wrong reason if you think he is difficult, and the very difficulty becomes an attraction. Somebody asked Edmund Hillary, who conquered the Everest—the highest peak, the only peak which was unconquered—somebody asked, "Why? Why you take such trouble? What is the need? And even if you reach to the peak, what you will do? You will have to come back."

Said Hillary that, "It is a challenge to the human ego. An unconquered peak has to be conquered!" No other utility. . . What you will do? What he has done? He went there and put a flag and came back. What nonsense! And many people died in this effort. Almost for hundred years many groups had been trying. Many died, were lost, fell into the abyss, never came back, but the more it became difficult to reach, the more appeal.

Why go to moon? What will you do? Is not earth enough? But, no, the human ego cannot tolerate this—that the moon remains unconquered. Man must reach, because it is so difficult, it has to be conquered. So you can be attracted for wrong reasons. Now going to moon is not a poetic effort; it is not like small children who raise their hands and try to catch the moon.

Since humanity came into existence, every child has longed to reach to the moon. Every child has tried, but the difference must be understood deeply. The effort of a child is beautiful. The moon is so beautiful. It is a poetic effort to touch it, to reach it. There is no ego. It is a simple attraction, a love affair. Every child falls in that love affair. If you can find a child who is not attracted by the moon, what type of child is that?

Moon creates a subtle poetry, a subtle attraction. One would like to touch it and feel it; one would like to go to the moon. But that is not the reason for the scientist. For the scientist the moon is there, a challenge. How this moon dares to be there continuously, to be a challenge, and man is here and he cannot reach! He has to reach.

You can be attracted for wrong reasons. The fault is not with moon, neither the fault will be with Patanjali. But you should not be attracted for wrong reasons. Patanjali is difficult—the most difficult—because he analyzes the whole path, and each fragment seems to be very difficult, but difficulty should not be the appeal—remember that. You can walk through Patanjali's door, but you should fall in love not with the difficulty, but with the insight—the light that Patanjali throws on the path. You should fall in love with the light, not with the difficulty of the path. That will be a wrong reason.

*What you have been saying about Heraclitus, Christ and Zen seems like kindergarten teachings compared to Patanjali.*

And please don't compare. Comparison is also out of the ego. In real existence, things exist without any comparison. A tree which reaches four hundred feet into the sky, and a very, very small grass flower are both the same as far as existence is concerned. But you go and you say, "This is a great tree. And what is this? Just ordinary grass." You bring the comparison in, and wherever comparison comes, comes ugliness. You have destroyed a beautiful phenomenon.

The tree was great in its "tree-ness" and the grass was great in its "grassiness". The tree may have risen four hundred feet. Its flowers may flower in the highest sky, and the grass is just clinging to the earth. Its flowers will be very, very small. Nobody may be even aware when they flower and when they fade. But when this grass flowers, the phenomenon of flowering is the same, the celebration is the same, and there is not a bit of difference. Remember this: that in existence there is no comparison; mind brings the comparison. It says, "You are more beautiful." Can't you simply say, "You are beautiful"? Why bring "more"?

Mulla Nasruddin was in love with a woman, and as women are prone to ask, the woman asked, when Mulla Nasruddin kissed her, "Are you kissing me the first woman? Am I the first woman whom you are kissing? Is your first kiss given to a woman?" Nasruddin said, "Yes, the first and the most sweetest."

Comparison is in your blood. You cannot remain with a thing as it is. The woman is also asking for a comparison; otherwise why be worried about whether this is a first kiss or a second? Each kiss is fresh and virgin. It has no relationship with any other kiss of the past or of the future. Each kiss is an existence in itself. It exists alone in its solitariness. It is a peak in itself; it is a unit—not in any way connected with the past or with the future. Why ask whether it is the first? And what beauty the first carries? And why not the second, and why not the third?

But the mind wants to compare. Why the mind wants to compare? Because through comparison ego is fed, that "I am the first woman; this is the first kiss." You are not interested in the kiss—in the quality of the kiss. This moment the kiss opened a door of heart; you are not interested in that, that is nothing. You are interested in whether it is a first or not. The ego is always interested in comparison, and existence knows no comparison. And people like Heraclitus, Patanjali, they live in existence, not in mind. Don't compare them.

Many people come to me and they say that, "Who is great, Buddha or Christ?" What foolishness to ask! "Buddha is greater than Christ and Christ is greater than Buddha," I say to them; "Why you go on comparing?" A subtle thing is there working. If you are a follower of Christ, you would like Christ to be the greatest because you can only be great if Christ is the greatest. It is a fulfillment of your own ego. How can your Master not be the greatest? He has to be because you are such a great disciple. And if Christ is not the greatest, then where Christians will be? If Buddha is not the greatest, then what will happen to the ego of the Buddhists?

Every race, every religion, every country, thinks itself to be the greatest — not because any country is great, not because any race is great: in this existence everything is the greatest. The existence creates only the greatest, every being unique. But that doesn't appeal to the mind because then greatness is so common. Everybody great? Then what is the use of it! Somebody has to be lower. A hierarchy has to be created.

Just the other night, I was reading a book of George Mikes, and he said that in Budapest, in Hungary, where he is born, one English woman fell in love with him. In Hungary, an English woman fell in love with him. But he was not much in love; but he didn't want to be rude also, so when she asked that, "Can we not get married?" he said, "It will be difficult because my mother will not allow me, and will not be happy if I marry a foreigner." The English lady was very much offended. She said, "What? I and a foreigner? I am not a foreigner! I am English! You are a foreigner and your mother too!"

Mikes said that, "In Budapest, in Hungary, I am a foreigner?" The woman said, "Yes! Truth does not depend on geography."

Everybody thinks that way. The mind tries to fulfill its desires, to be the most suprememost. From religion, race, country, everything, one has to be watchful—very watchful. Only then you can get beyond this subtle phenomenon of the ego.

*Heraclitus, Christ and Zen make the final step*
*seem close; Patanjali makes even the first step*
*seem almost impossible.*

—because it is both. "He is closer than the closest and he is farther than the farthest," says the Upanishad. He is both near and far. He has to be, because who will be far then? And he has to be near also, because who will be near you? He touches your skin, and he is spread beyond the boundaries. He is both!

Heraclitus emphasizes the nearness because he is a simple man. And he says that he is so near, nothing is needed to do to bring him nearer. He is almost there; he is just watching at the gate, knocking at your door, waiting near your heart. Nothing is to be done. You simply be silent and have a look; just sit silently and look. You have never lost him. The truth is near.

In fact, to say it is near is wrong because you are also truth. Even nearness seems to be very, very far; even nearness shows that there is a distinction, a distance, a gap. Even that gap is not there: you are it! Says the Upanishad, "Thou art that: *Tattwamasi Swetaketu.*" You are already that: even that much distance is not there to say that he is close.

Because Heraclitus and Zen they want you to take the jump immediately—not wait. Patanjali says he is very far. He is also right: he is very far also. And he will appeal you more, because if he is so close and you have not attained him, you will feel very, very depressed. If he is so close, just by the side of the corner, just standing by the side of you, if he is the only neighbor, and from everywhere he surrounds you and you have not achieved, your ego will feel very very frustrated. Such a great man like you, and he is so near and you are missing? That seems very frustrating. But if he is very far, then everything is okay because time is needed, effort is needed—nothing is wrong with you, he is so far away.

Distance is such a vast thing. You will take time, you will go, you will move, and one day you will achieve. If he is near, then you will feel guilty. Then why you are not achieving him? Reading Heraclitus and Basho and Buddha, one feels uncomfortable. Never that happens with Patanjali. One feels at ease.

Look at the paradox of the mind. With the easiest of people one feels uncomfortable. Uncomfort comes from you. To move with Heraclitus or Jesus is very uncomfortable because they go on insisting that the kingdom of God is within you, and you know that nothing exists except hell within you. And they insist the kingdom of God is within you; it becomes uncomfortable.

If the kingdom of God is within you, the something is wrong with you. Why you cannot see it? And if it is so present, why not it can happen right this moment? That is the message of Zen—that it is immediate. There is no need to wait, no need to waste time. It can happen right now, this very moment. There is no excuse. This makes uncomfortable; you feel uncomfortable, you cannot find any excuse. With Patanjali millions of excuses you can find, that he is very far. Millions of lives effort is needed. Yes, it can be attained, but always in the future. You are at ease. There is no urgency about it, and you can be as you are right now. Tomorrow morning you will start moving on the path, and the tomorrow never comes.

Patanjali gives you space, future. He says, "Do this and that and that, and by and by you will reach—some day, nobody knows—in some future life." You are at ease, no urgency. You can be as you are; there is no hurry.

These Zen people, they drive you crazy, and I drive you more crazy, Mm?—because I talk from both the sides. This is just a way. This is a koan. This is just a way to drive you crazy. Heraclitus I use, Patanjali I use, but these are tricks to drive you crazy. You simply cannot be allowed to relax. Whenever there is future, you are okay. Then the mind can desire God, and nothing is wrong with you. The very phenomenon is such that it will take time. This becomes an excuse.

With Patanjali you can postpone; with Zen you cannot postpone. If you postpone, it is you who are postponing, not God. With Patanjali you can postpone, because the very nature of God is such that it can be attained only in gradual ways. Very, very difficult, that's why with difficulty you feel comfortable, and this is the paradox: people who say it is easy, you feel uncomfortable; people who say difficult, you feel comfortable. It should be just the otherwise.

And the truth is both, so it depends on you. If you want to postpone, Patanjali is perfect. If you want it here and now, then you will have to listen to Zen and you will have to decide. Are you in an urgency? Have you not suffered enough? Do you want to suffer more? Then Patanjali is perfect. You follow Patanjali. Then somewhere in the distant future you will attain to bliss. But if you have suffered enough—and this is what maturity is: to understand that you have suffered enough.

And you call Heraclitus and Zen for children? Kindergarten? This is the only maturity, to have realized that, "I have suffered enough." If you feel this, then an urgency is created, then a fire is created. Something has to be done right now! You cannot postpone it; there is no meaning in postponing. You have postponed it already enough. But if you want future, you would like to suffer a little more, you have become addicted with the hell, just one day more to remain the same, or you would like some modifications. . .

That's what Patanjali says: "Do this, do that, slowly. Do one thing, then another thing," and millions of things have to be done, and they cannot be done immediately, so you go on modifying yourself. Today you take a vow that you will be non-violent; tomorrow you will take another vow. Then day after tomorrow you will become a celibate, and this way it goes on and on, and then there are millions of things to be left: lying is to be dropped, violence is to be dropped, aggression is to be dropped; anger, hate, jealousy, possessiveness — millions of things you have — by and by. And meanwhile you remain the same.

How can you drop anger if you have not dropped hate? How can you drop anger if you have not dropped jealousy? How can you drop anger if you have not dropped aggressiveness? They are interrelated. So you say that now you will no more be angry, but what are you talking? Nonsense! Because you will remain hateful, you will remain aggressive, you will like to dominate, you love to be at the top, and you are dropping anger? How you can drop it? They are interrelated.

This is what Zen says: that if you want to drop, understand the phenomenon that everything is related. Either you drop it now, or you never drop it. Don't befool. You can simply whitewash: a little here, a patch there, and the old house remains with all its oldness. And while you go on working, painting the walls and filling the holes and this and that, you think you are creating a new life, and meanwhile you continue the same. And the more you continue, the more it becomes deep-rooted.

Don't deceive. If you can understand, understanding is immediate. That is the message of Zen. If you cannot understand, then something has to be done, and Patanjali will be good. You follow Patanjali. One day or other, you will have to come to an understanding where you will see that this whole thing has been a trick — trick of your mind to avoid, to avoid the reality, to avoid and escape — and that day suddenly you will drop.

Patanjali is gradual, Zen is sudden. If you cannot be sudden, then it is better to be gradual. Rather than being nothing, neither this nor that, it is better you be gradual. Patanjali will also bring you to the same situation, but he will give you a little space. It is more comfortable — difficult, but more comfortable. No immediate transformation is demanded, and with gradual progress, mind can fit.

> Heraclitus, Christ and Zen make the final step
> seem close; Patanjali makes even the first step
> seem almost impossible. It seems like us
> westerners have hardly begun to realize the
> amount of work that has to be done.

It is up to you. If you want to do the work, you can do. If you want to realize without doing the work, that too is possible. That too is possible! It is up to you to choose! If you want to do hard work, I will give you hard work. I can create even more steps. Patanjali can be made even more long, stretched. I can put the goal even farther away; I can give you impossible things to do. It is your choice. Or if you want really to realize, then this can be done this very moment. It is up to you. Patanjali is a way of looking, Heraclitus is also a way of looking.

Once it happened: I was passing through the street and I saw a small child eating a very big watermelon. The melon was too big for him, and I looked and I watched and I saw that he is finding a little difficulty to finish. So I asked him, I told him, "It seems to be really too big; isn't it so?" The boy looked at me and said, "No! Not enough me."

He is also right. Everything can be looked from two standpoints. God is near and far. Now it is for you to decide from where you would like to take the jump —

from the near or from the far. If you want to take the jump from the far, then come all the techniques, because they will take you far, from there you will take the jump. It is just like you are standing on this shore of the ocean; the ocean is here also and there at the other shore also—which is completely invisible, very, very far away. You can take the jump from this shore because it is the same ocean, but if you decide to take the jump from the other shore Patanjali gives you a boat.

The whole yoga is a boat to go to the other shore, to take the jump. It is up to you. You can enjoy the journey; there is nothing wrong in it. I am not saying it is wrong. It is up to you. You can take the boat and go to the other shore, and take the jump from there. But the same ocean exists. Why not take from this shore? The jump will be the same, and the ocean will be the same, and you will be the same. What difference does it make to go to the other shore? There may be people on the other shore, and they may be trying to come here. There are also Patanjalis; they have made boats there. They are coming towards here to take the jump from the faraway.

It happened: one man was trying to cross a road. And it was a peak hour, and it was difficult to cross the road; so many cars going so fast, and he was a very, very mild man. He tried many times and then came back. Then he saw Mulla Nasruddin on the other side —old acquaintance. He cried, "Nasruddin, how you crossed the road?" Nasruddin said, "I never crossed. I was born on this side."

There are people who are always thinking of the distant shore. The distant always looks beautiful, the distant has a magnetism of its own, because it is covered in mist. But the ocean is the same. It is up to you to choose. Nothing is wrong, going to that ocean, but go for right reasons. You may be simply avoiding the jump from this shore. Then even if the boat leads you to the other shore, the moment you reach the other shore you will start thinking of this shore, because then this will be the faraway point. And many times, in many lives, you have done this. You have changed the shore, but you have not taken the jump.

I have seen you crossing the ocean from this side to that and from that side to this. Because this is the problem: that shore is far away because you are here; when you will be there, this shore will be far away. And you are in such a sleep that you completely forget again and again that you have been to that shore also. By the time you reach to the other shore, you have forgotten the shore that you have left behind. By the time you reach, oblivion takes over.

You look to the distant, and again somebody says, "Here is a boat, sir. You can go to the other shore, and you can take the jump from there because God is very, very far away." And you again start preparation to leave this shore. Patanjali gives you a boat to go to the other, but when you have reached to the other, Zen will give you always the jump. The final jump is of the Zen. Meanwhile you can do many things; that is not the point. Whenever you will take the jump it will be a sudden jump. It cannot be gradual!

All "gradualness" is going from this shore to that. But nothing is wrong in it. If you enjoy the journey it is beautiful, because he is here, he is in the middle, he is at that shore also. No need to reach to the other shore either. You can take the jump in the middle also, just from the boat. Then boat becomes the shore. From where you jump is the shore. Every moment you can take the jump; then it becomes the shore. If you don't take the jump, then it is no more the shore. It depends on you; remember this well.

That's why I am talking about all contradictory standpoints, so that you can understand from everywhere and you can see the reality from everywhere and then you can decide. If you decide to wait a little, beautiful. If you decide to take right now, beautiful. To me, everything is beautiful and great, and I have no choice. I simply give you all the choices. If you say, "I would like to wait a little," I say, "Good! I bless you. Wait a little." If you say, "I am ready and I want to jump," I say, "Jump, with my blessings."

For me there is no choice — neither Heraclitus, nor Patanjali. I am simply opening all the doors for you with the hope that you may enter some door. But remember the tricks of the mind. When I talk about Heraclitus, you think it is too vague, too mysterious, too simple. When I talk about Patanjali, you think it is too difficult, almost impossible. I open the door, and you interpret something and take a judgment and you stop yourself. The door is open not for you to judge. The door is open for you to enter.


The second question:

*You talked of moving from faith to trust. How can we use the mind that swings from doubt to belief to go beyond these two polarities?*

Doubt and belief are not different — two aspects of the same coin. This has to be understood first, because people think that when they believe, they have gone beyond doubt. Belief is the same as doubt because both are mind concern. Your mind argues, says no, finds no proof to say yes; you doubt. Then your mind finds arguments to say yes, proofs to say yes, you believe. But in both the cases you believe in reason; in both the cases, you believe in arguments. The difference is just on the surface; deep down you believe in the reasoning, and trust is dropping out of reasoning. It is mad! It is irrational! It is absurd!

And I say trust is not faith; trust is a personal encounter. Faith again is given and borrowed. It is a conditioning. Faith is a conditioning parents, culture, society give you. You don't bother about it; you don't make it a personal concern. It is a given thing, and which is given and which has not been a personal growth, is just a facade, a false face, a Sunday face.

On six days you are different; you enter church and you put on a mask. See how people behave in church; so gently, so humanly—the same people! Even a murderer comes to church and prays, see the face—it looks so beautiful and innocent, and this man has killed. In church you have a proper face to use, and you know how to use it. It has been a conditioning. From the very childhood it has been given to you.

Faith is given; trust is a growth. You encounter reality, you face reality, you live reality, and by and by you come to an understanding that doubt leads to hell, misery. The more you doubt, the more miserable you become. If you can doubt completely, you will be in a perfect misery. If you are not in a perfect misery, that is because you cannot doubt completely. You still trust. Even an atheist, he also trusts. Even a man who doubts whether the world exists or not, he also trusts; otherwise he cannot live, life will become impossible.

If doubt becomes total, you cannot live a single moment. How can you breathe in if you doubt? If you really doubt, who knows the breath is not poisonous! Who knows millions of germs are not being carried into! Who knows cancer is not coming through the breath! If you really doubt, you cannot even breathe. You cannot live a single moment; you will die immediately. Doubt is suicide. But you never doubt perfectly, so you linger on. You linger on; you somehow drag on. But your life is not total. Just think: if total doubt is suicide, then total trust will be the absolute life possible.

That's what happens to a man of trust: he trusts, and the more he trusts, the more he becomes capable to trust. The more he becomes capable of trust, the more life opens. He feels more, he lives more, he lives intensely. Life becomes an authentic bliss. Now he can trust more. Not that he is not deceived, because if you trust, that doesn't mean that nobody is going to deceive you. In fact, more people will deceive you because you become vulnerable. If you trust, more people will deceive you, but nobody can make you miserable; that's the point to understand. They can deceive, they can steal things from you, they can borrow money and they will never return — but nobody can make you miserable — that becomes impossible. Even if they kill you, they cannot make you miserable.

You trust, and trust makes you vulnerable — but absolutely victorious also, because nobody can defeat you. They can deceive, they can steal, you may become a beggar, but still you will be an emperor. Trust makes emperors out of beggars and doubt makes beggars out of emperors. Look at an emperor, who cannot trust; he is always afraid. He cannot trust his own wife, he cannot trust his own children, because a king possesses so much that the son will kill him, the wife will poison him. He cannot trust anybody. He lives in such a distrust, he is already in hell. Even if he sleeps, he cannot relax. Who knows what's going to happen!

Trust makes you more and more open. Of course, when you are open, many things will become possible. When you are open, friends will reach to your heart; of course, enemies can also reach to your heart — the door is open. So there are two possibilities. If you want to be secure, you close the door completely. Bolt it, lock it and hide within. Now no enemy can enter, but no friend can enter also. Even if God comes, he cannot enter. Now nobody can deceive you, but what is the point? You are in a grave. You are already dead. Nobody can kill you, but you are already dead; you cannot come out. You live in security, of course, but what type of life is this? You don't live at all. Then you open the door.

Doubt is closing the door; trust is opening the door. When you open the door, all the alternatives become possible. Friend may enter, foe may enter. Wind will come; it will bring the perfume of the flowers; it will also bring the germs of diseases. Now everything is possible — the good and bad. Love will come; hate will also come. Now God can come, devil can also come. This is the fear that something may go wrong, so close the door. But then everything goes wrong. Open the door — something is possible to go wrong, but for you, nothing, if your trust is total. Even in the enemy you will find the friend and even in the devil you will find God. Trust is such a transformation that you cannot find the bad because your whole outlook has changed.

That is the meaning of Jesus' saying, "Love your enemies." How can you love your enemies? It has been a problem to be solved — an enigma for Christian theologians. How can you love your enemy? But a man of trust can do, because a man of trust knows no enemies. A man of trust knows only the friend. In whatsoever form he comes makes no difference. If he comes to steal he is the friend; if he comes to take he is the friend; if he comes to give he is the friend: in whatsoever form he comes.

It happened that Al-Hillaj Mansoor, a great mystic, a great Sufi, was murdered, killed, crucified. The last of his words were — he looked at the sky — and he said, "But you cannot deceive me." Many people were there, and Al-Hillaj was smiling, and he said towards the sky, "Look, you cannot deceive me." So somebody asked, "What do you mean? To whom you are talking?" He said, "I am talking to my God: in whatsoever form you come you cannot deceive me. I know you well. Now you have come as death. You cannot deceive me."

A man of trust cannot be deceived. In whatsoever form, whosoever comes, it is always the divine coming to him because trust makes everything holy. Trust is an alchemy. It transforms not only you; it transforms for you the whole world. Wherever you look you find him: in the friend, in the foe; in the night, in the day. Yes, Heraclitus is right. God is summer and winter, day and night; God is satiety and hunger. This is trust. Patanjali makes trust the base — the base of all growth.

*You talked of moving from faith to trust. . .*

Faith is that which is given; trust is that which is found. Faith is given by your parents; trust has to be found by you. Faith is given by the society; trust you have to search and seek and inquire. Trust is personal, intimate; faith is like a commodity. You can purchase it in the market.

You can purchase it in the market — when I say it, I say it with a very considered mind. You can go and become a Mohammedan; you can go and become a Hindu. Go in an Arya temple and you can be converted to be a Hindu. There is no difficulty. Faith can be purchased in the market. From Mohammedan you can become Hindu, from Hindu you can become Jain. It is so simple that any foolish priest can do it. But trust — it is not a commodity. You cannot go and find it in the market; you cannot purchase it. You have to pass through many experiences. By and by it arises; by and by it changes you. A new quality, a new flame comes to your being.

When you see that doubt is misery, then comes trust. When you see faith is dead, then comes trust. You are a Christian, Hindu, Mohammedan; have you ever observed that you are completely dead? What type of Christian you are? If you are really a Christian, you will be a Christ — nothing less than that. Trust will make you Christ, faith will make you a Christian — a very poor substitute. What type of Christian you are? Because you go to the church, because you read the Bible? Your faith is not a knowing. It is an ignorance.

It happened in a Rotary Club somewhere: a great economist came to talk. He talked in the jargon of the economics. The priest of the town was also present to listen to him. After the talk, he came to him and said, "It was a beautiful talk you gave, but to be frank, I couldn't follow a single word." The economist said, "In that case, I would say to you what you say to your listeners: have faith!"

When you cannot understand, when you are ignorant, the whole society says, "Have faith." I will say to you: it is better to doubt than to have a false faith. It is better to doubt, because doubt will create misery. Faith is a consolation; doubt will create misery. And if there is misery, you will have to seek trust. This is the problem, the dilemma that has happened in the world. Because of faith, you have forgotten how to seek trust. Because of faith you have become trustless. Because of faith you carry corpses: you are Christians, Hindus, Mohammedans, and you miss the whole point. Because of faith you think you are religious. Then the inquiry stops.

Honest doubt is better than dishonest faith. If your faith is false — and all faith is false if you have not grown into it, if it is not your feeling and your being and your experience — all faith is false! Be honest. Doubt! Suffer! Only suffering will bring you to understanding. If you suffer truly one day or other you will understand that it is doubt that is making me suffer. And then the transformation becomes possible.

> You ask me, *How can we use the mind that swings from doubt to belief to go beyond these two polarities?*

You cannot use it, because you have never been an honest doubter. Your faith is false: doubt is deep down hidden. Just on the surface a whitewash of faith is there. Deep down you are doubtful — but you are afraid to know that you are doubtful, so you go on clinging with faith, you go on making gestures of faith. You can make gestures, but through gestures you cannot attain to reality. You can go and bow down in a shrine; you are making the gesture of a man who trusts. But you will not grow, because deep down there is no trust, only doubt. Faith is just superimposed.

It is just like kissing a person you don't love. From the outside everything is the same; you are making the gesture of kissing. No scientist can find any difference. If you kiss a person, the photograph, the physiological phenomenon, the transfer of millions of germs from one lip to another, everything, exactly is the same whether you love or not. If a scientist watches and observes, what will be the difference? No difference — not even a single iota of difference! He will say both are kisses and exactly the same.

But you know when you love a person then something of the invisible passes which cannot be detected by any instrument. When you don't love a person, then you can give the kiss, but nothing passes. No energy communication, no communion happens. The same is with faith and trust. Trust is a kiss with love, with a deeply loving heart, and faith is a kiss without any love.

So from where to begin? The first thing is to inquire into the doubt. Throw the false faith. Become an honest doubter — sincere. Your sincerity will help, because if you are honest how can you miss the point that doubt creates suffering? If you are sincere, you are bound to know. Sooner or later you will come to realize that doubt has been creating more misery — the more you go into doubt, the more misery. And only through misery one grows.

And when you come to a point where misery becomes impossible to tolerate, intolerable, you drop it. Not that really you drop it; the very intolerability becomes the drop. And once there is not doubt and you have suffered through it, you start moving towards trust.

Trust is transformation — *shraddha*; and, says Patanjali, that *shraddha* — trust — is the base of all *samadhi*, of all ultimate experience of the divine.

# Total Effort Or Surrender

*Success is nearest to those whose efforts are intense and sincere.*

*The chances of success vary according to the degree of effort.*

*Success is also attained by those who surrender to God.*

*God is the supreme ruler. He is an individual unit of of divine consciousness. He is untouched by the afflictions of life, action and its result.*

*In God the seed is developed to its highest extent.*

HERE ARE THREE TYPES OF seekers. The first type comes onto the path because of curiosity: Patanjali calls it *kutuhal*. He is not really interested. He has drifted into it as if by accident. He may have read something. He may have heard somebody talk about God, the truth, the ultimate liberation, and he became interested.

The interest is intellectual, just like a child who becomes interested in everything and each thing and then, after a time, drifts away because more and more curiosities are always opening their doors.

Such a man will never attain. Out of curiosity you

cannot attain the truth, because truth needs a persistent effort, a continuity, a perseverance which a man of curiosity cannot do. A man of curiosity can do a certain thing for a certain period of time according to his mood, but then there is a gap and in that gap all that is made disappears, is unmade. Again he will start from the very beginning, and the same will happen.

He cannot crop the result. He can sow the seeds; but he cannot wait, because millions of new interests are always calling him. He goes to the south, then he moves to the east, then he goes to the west, then to the north. He is like a drifting wood in the sea. He is not going anywhere; his energy is not moving to a certain goal. Whatsoever circumstance pushes him. . . Accidental he is and the accidental man cannot attain to the divine. And he may do much activity, but it is all futile because in the day he will make and in the night he will unmake it. A perseverance is needed; a continuous hammering is needed.

Jalaludin Rumi had a small school — a school of wisdom. He used to take his disciples to the fields, to the farms around. Particularly one farm he used to take all his new disciples to show what has happened there. Whenever a new disciple will come, he will take him to that farm. There was something worth. The farmer was an example of a certain state of mind. The farmer was digging a well, but he will dig ten feet, fifteen feet, and then he will change the mind. "This place doesn't look good" — so he will start another hole and then another.

Since many years, he has been doing that. Now there were eight incomplete holes. The whole farm was destroyed, and he was working on the ninth. Jalaludin will say to his new disciples, "Look! Don't be like this farmer. If he had put all his effort into one hole, by this time the hole would have been one hundred feet at least. He has made much effort; much activity he has done, but he cannot wait. Ten, twelve, fifteen feet, then he gets bored. Then he starts another hole. This way the whole farm will be covered with holes, and there will never be a well."

This is the man of curiosity, the accidental man who does things, and when he starts, he has much zeal — in fact, too much. And this too much zeal cannot become a continuity. He starts with such vigor and zest that you know that soon he will stop.

The second type of man who comes to the inner search is the man of *jigyasa* — inquiry. He has not come out of curiosity. He has come with an intense inquiry. He means it, but he is also not enough because his meaning is basically intellectual. He may become a philosopher, but he cannot become a religious man. He will inquire deeply, but his inquiry is intellectual. It remains head-oriented; it is a problem to be solved.

Life and death is not involved; it is not a question of life and death. It is a riddle, a puzzle. He enjoys solving it just as you enjoy solving a crossword puzzle because it gives you a challenge. It has to be solved, you will feel very good if you can solve it. But this is intellectual, and deep down ego is involved. This man will become a philosopher. He will try hard. He will think, contemplate, but he will never meditate. He will reflect logically, rationally; he will find many clues. He will create a system, but the whole thing will be his own projection.

Truth needs you totally. Even ninety-nine percent won't do: exactly hundred percent of you is needed, and head is only one percent. You can live without the head. Animals are living without the head, trees are living without the head. Head is not such an essential thing in existence. You can easily live — in fact, you can more easily live without the head than you are living with the head. It creates millions of complexities. Head is not just an absolute necessity and nature knows that. It is a superfluous luxury. If you have not enough food, the body knows where the food should go: it stops giving it to the head.

That's why, in poor countries, intellect cannot de-
velop, because intellect is a luxury. When everything is
finished, when the body is completely getting everything, only then the energy moves towards the head.
Even in your life it happens every day, but you are not
aware. Eat too much food—immediately you feel
sleepy. What is happening? The body needs energy to
digest. The head can be forgotten; the energy moves
towards the stomach. Head feels dizzy, sleepy. Energy is
not moving, blood is not moving, towards head. The
body has its own economy.

There are basic things, there are non-basic things.
Basic things have to be fulfilled first, because the non-
basic can wait, your philosophy can wait. There is not
much necessity for it. But your stomach cannot wait.
Your stomach has to be fulfilled first; that hunger is
more basic. Because of this basic realization many
religions have tried fasting, because if you fast the head
cannot think, because the energy is not so much; it
cannot be given to the head. But this is a deception.
When the energy will be there, the head will start thinking again. This meditation is a lie.

If you fast long, for few days continuously, the head
cannot think. Not that you have attained to no-mind;
simply superfluous energy doesn't exist in you now. The
body needs first; bodily needs are basic, essential; head
needs are secondary, superfluous. It is just as you have
an economy in your home. If your child is dying you
will sell the TV set. There is nothing much involved in
it. You can sell the furniture when the child is dying;
when you are hungry, you can sell even the house. First
things first—that is the meaning of economy—second
things second. And head is the last; it is only one percent of you, and that too superfluous. You can exist
without it.

Can you exist without the stomach? Can you exist
without the heart? But you can exist without the head.
And when you pay too much attention to the head, you

are completely upside down. You are doing *shirsha-sana*: standing on the head. You have completely forgotten that head is not essential.

And when you give only head to an inquiry, it is *jigyasa*. Then it is a luxury. You can become a philosopher and sit on an armchair; rest and think. Philosophers are like luxurious furniture. If you can afford, good, but it is not a life-and-death problem. So Patanjali says the man of *kutuhal* — the man of curiosity — cannot achieve; the man of *jigyasa* — inquiry — will become a philosopher.

Then there is the third man whom Patanjali calls the man of *mumuksha*. This word *mumuksha* is difficult to translate, so I will explain it. *Mumuksha* means the desire to be desireless, the desire to be completely liberated, the desire to get out of the wheel of existence, the desire not to be born again, not to die again, the feeling that it is enough — born millions of times, dying again and again and moving in the same vicious circle. *Mumuksha* means to become the ultimate drop-out from the very wheel of existence. Bored, suffering, and one wants to get out of it. The inquiry becomes now a life-and-death problem. Your whole being is at stake. Patanjali says only a man of *mumuksha*, to whom the desire for *moksha* — liberation — has arisen, can become a religious man, and then too because he is a very, very logical thinker.

Then too there are three types of men who belong to the category of *mumuksha*. The first type of man who belongs to *mumuksha* puts his one-third being into the effort. Putting one-third of your being into the effort, you will attain something. What you will attain will be a negative achievement: you will not be tense — this has to be understood very deeply — but, you will not be calm. You will not be tense; the tensions will drop. But you will not be tranquil, calm, cool. The attainment will be negative. You will not be ill, but you will not be healthy also. Illness will disappear. You will not feel irritated, you will not feel frustrated. But you will not feel fulfilled also. The negative will drop, the thorns will drop, but the flower has not come.

This is the first degree of *mumuksha*. You can find many people who are stuck there. You will feel a certain quality in them: they don't react, they don't get irritated, you cannot make them angry, you cannot put them in anxiety. They have attained something, but still you feel something is lacking. They are not at ease. Even non-angry, they don't have compassion. They may not be angry at you, but they cannot forgive. Subtle is the difference. They are not angry, that is right. But even in their being non-angry there is no forgiveness. They are stuck.

They don't bother about you, your insult, but they are, in a way, cut off from relationship. They can't share. Trying to be not angry, they have moved out of all relationships. They have become like islands— closed. And when you are an island, closed, you are uprooted. You cannot flower, you cannot be happy, you cannot have a well-being. It is a negative achievement. Something has been thrown, but nothing has been attained. The path is clear, of course. Even to throw something is very good because now the possibility comes into existence: you can attain something.

Patanjali calls them *mridu*: soft. The first degree of attainment, negative. You will find many sannyasins in India, many monks in Catholic monasteries, who are stuck at the first degree. They are good people, but you will find them dull. It is very good not to be angry, but it is not enough. Something is missing; nothing positive has happened. They are empty vessels. They have emptied themselves, but somehow they have not been refilled. The higher has not descended, but the lower has been thrown.

Then there is a second degree of *mumuksha*—the second degree of the right seeker—who puts himself two-thirds into the effort. Not yet total, just in the

middle. Because of the middle, Patanjali calls him
*madhya*—the middle man. He attains something. The
first-degree man is in him, but something more is added.
He is at peace—silent, cool, collected. Whatsoever
happens in the world does not affect him. He remains
unaffected, detached. He becomes like a peak: very
peaceful.

If you come near him you will feel his peace surrounding you; just as you go in a garden and the cool air
and the fragrance of the flowers and the singing of the
birds all surround you, they touch you, you can feel.
With the first-degree man, the *mridu*, you will not feel
anything. You will feel only an emptiness—a desert-like
being. And the first type of man will suck you. If you go
near him you will feel that you have been emptied—
somebody has been sucking you because he is a desert.
With him you will feel being dried, and you will be
afraid.

You will feel this with many sannyasins. If you go
near them, you will feel they are sucking you, not
knowingly. They have attained the first degree. They
have become empty, and that very emptiness becomes
like a hole and you are sucked by it automatically.

It is said in Tibet that this first-degree man, if he is
anywhere, should not be allowed to move in the town.
When lamas in Tibet attain to the first degree, they are
prohibited to go out of the monasteries—because if this
man comes near anybody, he sucks. That sucking is
beyond his control; he cannot do anything about it. He
is like a desert. Anything that comes near becomes
sucked, exploited.

It is not allowed for the first-degree lamas to touch a
tree because it has been observed that the tree dies. Even
in the Himalayas, a Hindu sannyasin is not allowed to
touch trees—they will die. He is a sucking phenomenon.
This first-degree lama is not allowed to attend anybody's marriage because he will become a destructive
force. He is not allowed to bless anybody because he

cannot bless. Even when he is blessing, he is sucking.
You may not have known it, for these first-degree
lamas, sannyasins, sadhus, monasteries were created, so
they can live in an enclosed world of their own, not
allowed to move out. Unless they attain to the second
degree, they are not allowed to bless anybody.

The second-degree seeker who has put his two-third
being becomes peaceful, calm. If you go near him, he
flows in you, he shares. Now he is no more a desert;
now he is a green forest. Many things are coming up in
him — silent, calm, tranquil. You will feel it. But this is
also not the goal; many are stuck there. Just to be silent
is not enough. What type of achievement is this? Just to
be silent? It is like death, no movement, no activity.
You are at peace of course, at home of course, but no
celebration, no bliss.

Third-degree seeker who puts his totality into it
attains to bliss. Bliss is a positive phenomenon; peace is
just on the way. When bliss comes nearer, you become
peaceful. It is a distant influence of the bliss that is
reaching near you. It is just like coming near a river:
from a long distance you start feeling that the air is
cooling, the quality of the greenery is changing. Trees
are greener with more foliage. The air is cool. The river
you have not seen yet, but the river is somewhere near,
the source of water is somewhere near. When the source
of life is somewhere near, you become peaceful, but you
have not attained yet — just on the way. Patanjali calls
this man the *madhya:* the middle man.

He is also not the goal. Unless you can dance with
ecstasy. . . This man cannot dance, this man cannot
sing, because singing will look like disturbing the peace,
dancing will look foolish — what are you doing? This
man can only sit like a dead statue — silent, of course,
but not flowering; green, but the flowers have not
happened yet: the final has not descended. Then there is
the third-degree man who can dance, who will look mad
because he has so much. He cannot contain and because

he cannot contain he will sing and he will dance and he will move and he will share, and he will throw wherever he can the seeds that are showering on him endlessly. This is the third-degree man.

Says Patanjali:

*Success is nearest to those whose efforts are intense and sincere.*

*The chances of success vary according to the degree of effort.*

*Success is nearest to those whose efforts are intense and sincere.* Your totality is needed. Remember, sincerity is a quality that happens whenever you are totally in something, but people are almost wrong in their idea of sincerity. They think to be serious is sincere. To be serious is not to be sincere. Sincerity is a quality which happens whenever you are totally in something. A child playing with his toys is sincere, totally in it, absorbed, nothing left behind, no holding back; he is not there really, only the play goes on.

Because if you don't hold anything, where you are? You have become completely one with the activity. The actor is no more there, the doer is no more there. When the doer is not, there is sincerity. How can you be serious? — because seriousness belongs to the doer. So in mosques, temples, churches, you will find two types of people — sincere and serious. Serious will be with long faces, as if they are doing a very great thing — something sacred, something of the other world. This too is ego, as if you are doing something great, as if you are obliging the whole world because you are praying.

Look at the religious people — so-called, of course: they walk in such a way as if they are obliging the whole world. They are the salt of the earth. If they disappear, the whole existence will disappear. They are supporting it. It is because of them life exists — because of their prayers. You will find them serious.

Seriousness belongs to the ego, the doer. Look at a father working in the shop, in the office somewhere. If he doesn't love his wife, his children, he will be serious because it is a duty. He is doing it, and he is obliging everybody around. He will always say, "I am doing it for my wife, I am doing it for my children." And this man by his seriousness will become a dead stone hanging around the necks of his children, and they will never be able to forgive this father because he never loved.

If you love, you never say such words. If you love your children, you go dancing to your office. You love them; it is not something that you are obliging. You are not fulfilling a duty; it is your love. You are happy that you are allowed to do something for your children. You are happy and blissful that you can do something for your wife because love feels so helpless; love wants to do so many things and cannot do. Love always feels that "Whatsoever I am doing is less than should be done." And duty? Duty always feels, "I am doing more than is needed." Duty becomes serious; love is sincere. And love is to be totally with a person, so totally to be with a person that the duality disappears — even for moments — there is no duality, one exists in two, a bridge comes in. Love is sincere, never serious. And wherever you can put your total being in anything, it becomes a love. If you are a gardener and you love, you bring your total being into it. Then sincerity happens.

Sincerity you cannot cultivate. Seriousness you can cultivate, but sincerity — no! Sincerity is a shadow of being total in something. Says Patanjali:

> Success is nearest to those whose efforts are
> intense and sincere.

Of course, there is no need to say intense and sincere. Sincerity is always intense. But why does Patanjali say intense and sincere? For a certain reason. Sincerity is always intense, but intensity is not necessarily always sincere. You can be intense in something but not sincere, may not be sincere. Hence, he adds the qualification, intense *and* sincere, because you can be intense even in your seriousness. You can be intense even with your part being, you can be intense in a certain mood, you can be intense in your anger, you can be intense in your lust, you can be intense in millions of things and may not be sincere, because sincerity belongs when you are totally in it.

You can be intense in sex and you may not be sincere, because sex is not necessarily love. You may be very, very intense in your sexuality — but once sexuality is fulfilled, it is finished, the intensity gone. Love may not look so intense, but it is sincere — and because it is sincere, the intensity continues. In fact, if you are really in love it becomes a timelessness. It is always intense. And make a clear distinction: if you are intense without sincerity, you cannot be forever intense. Only momentarily you can be intense; when the desire arises you are intense. It is not really your intensity. It is enforced by the desire.

Sex arises. You feel a starvation, a hunger. The whole body, the whole bio-energy, needs a release; you become intense. But this intensity is not yours; it is nothing coming from your being. It is just enforced by the biological crust around you: it is a bodily enforcement on your being. It is not coming from the center. It is being forced from the periphery. You will be intense, and then sex fulfilled, the intensity gone, then you don't care about the woman.

Many women have told me that they feel cheated, they feel deceived, they feel used because whenever their husbands make love to them, in the beginning they feel so loving, so intense; they feel so happy. But the moment sex is finished they turn over and go to sleep. They didn't care at all what is happening to the woman. After you have made love, you even don't say goodbye. You don't thank; the woman feels used.

Your intensity is biological, bodily; it is nothing

coming from you. In sex intensity there is a foreplay, but no afterplay. The word doesn't exist really. I have seen thousands of books written on sex; the word "afterplay" doesn't exist. What type of love is this? Bodily need fulfilled, finished. The woman has been used; now you can throw her just as you use something and throw it — a plastic container — you use it and you throw it. Finished! When the desire will arise, then again you will look at the woman, and at that woman you are very intense.

No, Patanjali doesn't mean that type of intensity. I have taken sex to explain to you, because that is the only intensity that is left with you. There is no other example possible. You have become so lukewarm in your life, you exist on such a low level of energy, that there is no intensity. Somehow you go to the office. Just stand by the corner of the road when the people are rushing toward their offices; just watch their faces — sleepy.

Where going? Why going? It seems as if they don't have anywhere else to go, so they are going to the office. They cannot help it; because what they will do at home? So they are going to the office, bored, automata, robot-like, going because everybody is going to the office and it is time to go. And what to do if you don't want to go? Holidays become such a suffering, no intensity. Coming back — look people in the evening, coming back to the house, not knowing why they are going again, but nowhere else to go, somehow, dragging life. Lukewarm, a low-energy phenomenon.

That is why I have taken the example of sex — because I cannot find any other intensity in you. You don't sing, you don't dance, you don't have any intensity. You don't laugh, you don't weep. All intensity is gone. In sex, a little intensity exists; that too because of nature — not because of you.

Patanjali says "intense and sincere". Religion is really like sex — deeper than sex, higher than sex, holier than sex, but like sex. It is one individual meeting with the whole: it is a deep orgasm. You melt into the whole, you completely disappear. Prayer is like love. Yoga — in fact, the very word "yoga" means meeting, communion, meeting of the two — and such a deep and intense and sincere meeting that the two disappear. The boundaries become blurred and one exists. It cannot be in any other way. If you are not sincere and intense, bring your total being. Only then the ultimate is possible. You have to risk yourself completely; less than that won't do.

*The chances of success vary according to the degree of effort.*

This is one path — the path of will. Patanjali is basically concerned with the path of will, but he knows, he is aware, that the other path also exists, so he gives just a footnote.

That footnote is:

Ishwarapranidhanatwa: *Success is also attained by those who surrender to God.*

Just a footnote, just to indicate that the other path is also there. This is the path of will — effort intense, sincere, total. Bring your wholeness to it. But Patanjali is aware; all those who know, are aware. And Patanjali is very considerate, he is a very scientific mind; he will not leave a single loophole. But that is not his path, so he simply gives a footnote just to remember that the other path is there.

Ishwarapranidhanatwa: *Success is also attained by those who surrender to God.*

Effort or surrender, but the basic thing is the same: totality is needed. Paths differ, but they cannot differ absolutely. Their shape, their form, their direction, may differ, but their inner meaning and significance has to remain the same because both lead to the divine. Effort: your totality is needed. Surrender: again your totality is needed. So to me there is only one path, and that is: bring your totality.

Whether you bring it through effort — yoga — it is up to you, or you bring it through *samarpan* — surrender, let-go — it is up to you. But remember always that a totality will be needed; you have to stake yourself completely. It is a gambling — a gamble with the unknown. And nobody can say when it will happen — nobody can predict, nobody can give you a guarantee. You gamble. You may win, you may not win. The possibility of not winning is always there because it is a very complex phenomenon. It is not as simple as it looks. But if you go on gambling, it has to happen one day.

If you miss one time don't be depressed, because even a Buddha has to miss many times. If you miss, just get up and risk again. Some time, in some unknown manner, the whole existence culminates to help you. Some time and in some unknown way, you hit the target exactly the right time when the door was open. But you have to hit many times. You go on throwing your arrow of consciousness. Don't bother about the result. It is very dark and the goal is not fixed; it goes on changing. So you go on throwing your arrow in the dark. Many times you will miss, and I say to you so that you don't become depressed. Many times everybody misses, that is how it is. But if you go on and on and on and don't get depressed, it will happen. It has always happened. That's why infinite patience is needed.

What is surrender to God? How can you surrender? How surrender will become possible? That too becomes possible if you make many efforts, and you go on failing. You make many efforts, you depend on yourself; effort depends on oneself. It is a willpower — the path of will. You depend on yourself. You fail and you fail and you fail. You stand up, again you fall, you stand up again, and you again start walking. And then a moment comes, when you have been failing and failing and failing, and you come to see that your effort is the cause, because your effort has become your ego.

That is the problem on the path of will. Because a man who is working on the path of will — making efforts, methods, using techniques, doing this and that — is bound to accumulate a certain sense of "I am": "I am superior, special, extraordinary. I am doing this and that — austerities, fasting, *sadhana*. I have done this much."

On the path of will one has to be very, very watchful of the ego, because the ego is bound to come. If you can watch the ego, and you don't accumulate ego, there is no need to surrender — because if there is no ego, there is nothing to surrender. This has to be understood very, very deeply. And when you are understanding — trying to understand Patanjali — this is a very fundamental thing.

If you make your effort continuously for many lives, the ego is bound to arise. You have to be very watchful. You should work, you should make all efforts, but don't gather the ego. Then there is no need to surrender; you may hit the target without surrendering. There is no need because the disease doesn't exist.

If the ego is there, then the need arises to surrender. That's why Patanjali says — after talking about intense, sincere, total effort, he suddenly says —

Ishwarapranidhanatwa: *Success is also attained by those who surrender to God.*

If you feel continuously failing, then remember that the failure is not because of the divine. The failure is happening because of your ego, from where the arrow is being thrown, the source of your being, there something is happening — a diversion. Ego is collecting there. Then there is only one possibility: surrender it! You have failed with it so totally, in so many ways. You did this and that, you tried to do this and that, and you failed and failed and failed. When frustration becomes final and you cannot see what to do, Patanjali says, "Now surrender to God."

Patanjali is very rare in this sense. He does not believe in God; he is not a God-believer. God is also a technique. Patanjali doesn't believe in any God, that there is some God. No, he says God is a technique. Those who fail, for them this technique — the last. If you fail in that also, there is no way. Patanjali says it is not a question whether God exists or not; that is not the point at all. The point is that God is hypothetical. Without God it will be difficult to surrender. You will ask, "To whom?"

So God is a hypothetical point just to help surrender. When you have surrendered you will know there is no God, but that is when you have surrendered and when you have known. For Patanjali even God is a hypothesis to help you. It is a lie. That's why I told you Patanjali is a sly Master. It is just a help. Surrender is the basic thing, not God. And this difference you must note, because there are people who think God is the basic thing — because there is God you surrender.

Patanjali says that because you have to surrender, posit a God. God is a posited thing. When you have surrendered, you will laugh. There is no God! But one thing more: there are gods — no God — a multiplicity of gods, because whenever you surrender you become a god. So don't be confused with Patanjali's God and Christian-Jewish God. Patanjali says God is the potentiality of every being. Man is as if a seed of God — every man. And when the seed flowers, comes to a fulfillment, the seed has become a god. So every man, every being, will become finally a god.

"God" means just the ultimate culmination, the ultimate flowering. There is no God, but there are gods — infinite gods. This is a totally different conception. If you ask Mohammedans, they will say there is only one

God. If you ask Christians, they also say there is only one God. But Patanjali is more scientific. He says God is a possibility. Everybody is carrying that possibility within the heart. Everybody is just a seed, a potentiality to become a god. When you reach to the highest beyond which nothing exists, you become a god. Many have reached before you, many will reach — and many will be reaching after you.

Everyone becomes a god finally, because everyone is a god potentially, infinite gods. That is why it becomes difficult for Christians to understand. You call Rama a god, you call Krishna a god, you call Buddha a god, you call Mahavira a god. Even a Rajneesh you call a god.

For a Christian it becomes impossible to understand. What are you doing? For them only one God exists who has created the world. For Patanjali nobody has created the world. Millions of gods exist, and everybody is on the path to become a god. Whether you know it or not, you carry a god within your womb. And you may miss many times, but how can you miss it ultimately? If you carry it within you, some day or the other the seed is going to flower. You cannot miss it absolutely — no!

This is a totally different conception. Christian God seems to be very dictatorial, dominating the whole existence. Patanjali is more democratic — no despot, no dictator, no Stalin, no czar sitting on the top of the throne, with his only begotten son Christ by the side and the apostles around. This is nonsense. The whole concept is as if in the image of an emperor it has been made — on the throne. No, Patanjali is absolutely democratic. He says godliness is everybody's quality. You carry it; it is up to you to bring it to its totality. If you don't want it, that too is up to you.

Nobody is sitting as a despot on the world; nobody is forcing you or creating you. Freedom is absolute. You can sin because of freedom, you can move away because of freedom. You suffer because of freedom, and when you understand this, there is no need to suffer; you can come back, that too because of freedom. Nobody is bringing you back, and there is going to be no judgment day. Nobody is there to judge you except your own being. You are the doer, you are the judge, you are the criminal, you are the law. You are all! You are a miniature existence.

> *God is the supreme. He is an individual unit of divine consciousness.* Remember: *He is an individual unit of divine consciousness. He is untouched by the afflictions of life, action and its result.*

God is a state of consciousness. It is not a person, really, but "individual", so you will have to understand the difference between personality and individuality. Personality is the periphery. As you look to others, that is your personality. You say, "Nice personality, beautiful personality, ugly personality" — as you look to others. Your personality is the decision, the opinion of others about you. If you are alone on the earth, will you have any personality? No personality, because who will say you are beautiful, and who will say you are stupid, and who will say you are a great leader of men? There is nobody to say anything about you. The opinion will not be there, you will not have any personality.

The word personality comes from the Greek word "persona". In the Greek drama, the actors had to use masks. Those masks were called persona. From that persona comes the word personality. The face that you wear when you look at your wife and smile, that is personality — persona. You don't feel like smiling, but you have to smile. A guest comes and you welcome him, and deep down you never wanted him to come to you and deep down you are disturbed — "Now what to do with this man?" — but you are smiling and welcoming and you are saying that "So glad".

Personality is that which you pose, a face, a mask.

But if there is nobody in your bathroom, you don't have any personality unless you look in the mirror. Then immediately the personality comes because you yourself start doing the work of the other opinion. You look in the face and say, "Beautiful". Now you are divided, now you are two, giving opinion about yourself. But in the bathroom when nobody is there and you are completely unafraid, that nobody is looking from the keyhole. . . Because if somebody looks from the keyhole, personality comes in, you start behaving.

In the bathroom only you drop the personality. That's why bathroom is so refreshing. Out of the bath you come so beautiful, fresh, no personality; you become an individual. Individuality is that which you are; personality is that which you show that you are. Personality is your face; individuality is your being. God, in Patanjali's conception, has no personality. He is an individual unit.

If you grow, by and by, opinion of others becomes childish. You don't bother about them; what they say is meaningless. It is not what they say that carries meaning. It is you, what you are, that carries the meaning, not that they say, "Beautiful". This is useless. If you are beautiful, that is the point. What they say is irrelevant. What you are — the real, the authentic you — that is your individual.

When you drop personalities, you become a sannyasin. When you renounce personalities, you become a sannyasin: you become an individual unit. Now you live through your authentic center. You don't pose. When you don't pose, you are not worried. When you don't pose, you are unaffected by what others say. When you don't pose, you remain detached. Personality cannot remain detached. It is a very fragile thing. It exists between you and the other, and it depends on the other. He can change his mind; he can destroy you completely. You look at a woman and she smiles, and you feel so beautiful because of her smile. And if she simply turns with hatred in her eyes, you are simply crushed. In fact, you are crushed because your personality has been thrown under the shoes. She walked over you; she didn't look even.

Every moment you are afraid somebody may crush your personality. Then the whole world becomes an anxiety. A god has an individuality, but no personality. Whatsoever he is, that's what he shows. Whatsoever he is in, he is out. In fact, in and out have disappeared for him.

*God is the supreme.*

In English it is translated, *God is the supreme ruler.* That's why I say there exists a misunderstanding about Patanjali. In Sanskrit he calls him *purush-vishesh* — a supreme being, not a ruler. I will like to translate God as the supreme. He is an individual unit of divine consciousness — individual, remember, not universal, because Patanjali says every individual is a god.

*He is untouched by the afflictions of life, action, and its result.*

Why? Because the more you become individual, the more life takes a different quality. A new dimension opens — the dimension of play. The more you are concerned with the personality and the outer, the crust, the periphery. . . Your dimension of life is that of work: worried about the result, worried about whether you will attain the goal or not, always worried whether things are going to help you or not, what will happen tomorrow.

A man whose life has become a play is not worried about tomorrow, because he exists only today. Says Jesus, "Look at the lilies. They are so beautiful," because for them life is not a work. Look at rivers, look at stars. Except man, everything is beautiful and holy because the whole existence is a play. Nobody is worried about the result. Is the tree worried about whether flowers will come or not? Is the river worried whether she will reach to the ocean or not? Except man, there is no worry. Why man is worried? Because he looks life as work, not as play — and the whole existence is a play.

Says Patanjali: when one becomes centered into oneself, one becomes a player; he plays. Life is a game and it is beautiful; no need to worry about the result. Result doesn't matter, it is simply irrelevant. The thing which you are doing in itself has value. I am talking to you; you are listening to me. But you are listening with a purpose, and I am talking purposelessly. You are listening with a purpose, because through listening you are going to attain something — some knowledge, some clues, some techniques, methods, some understanding, and then you are going to work them out. You are after a result. I am talking to you purposelessly; I simply enjoy.

People ask me, "Why you go on talking every day?" I enjoy; it is just like birds singing. What is the purpose? Ask the rose why it goes on flowering? What is the purpose? I am talking to you because this sharing of myself with you is in itself a value, it has intrinsic value. I am not looking at the result; I am not worried whether you are transformed through it or not. There is no worry. If you listen me, that's all. And if you are also not worried, then transformation can happen this very moment. Because you are worried how to use it — whatsoever I say, how to use it — what to do about it. . .

You are already in the future. You are not here; you are not playing the game. You are in a workshop. You are not playing the game! You are thinking to gain some results out of it, and I am absolutely purposeless. It is how I share myself with you. I am talking not to do something in the future: I am talking because right now, through this sharing, something is happening, and that's enough.

Remember the words "intrinsic value", and make your every act an intrinsic value. Don't bother about the result—because the moment you think about the result, whatsoever you are doing becomes the means and the end is in the future. Make the means themselves the end; make the path the goal. Make this very moment the ultimate; there is no beyond it. This is the state of God and whenever you are playing, you have some glimpses of it.

Children play, and you cannot find anything diviner than children playing. Hence, Jesus says, "Unless you become like children, you will not enter into the kingdom of my God." Become like children. The meaning is not to become childish, because to be childish is totally a different thing; to be like children is totally a different thing. Childishness has to be dropped. That is juvenile, foolish. To be like children has to be increased. That is innocence—purposeless innocence. Profit brings the poison in; the result poisons you. Then innocence is lost.

*God is the supreme. He is an individual unit of divine consciousness. He is untouched by the afflictions of life, action and its result.*

You can become a god right now because you are already that—just the thing has to be realized. You are already the case. It is not that you have to grow into a god. Really, you have to realize that you are already that. This happens through surrender.

Patanjali says you believe in a God, you trust in a God there, somewhere, high in the universe, at the top, and you surrender. That God is just a prop to help surrender. When the surrender happens you become a god, because surrender means, "Now I am not concerned with the result, I am not concerned with the future, I am not concerned with myself at all. I surrender!"

When you say, "I surrender", what is surrender? I— the ego! And without the ego how can you think about purpose, result? Who will think about it? Then you are in a let-go. Then you go wherever it leads. Now the whole will decide; you have surrendered your decision. Patanjali says there are two ways. Make effort total. If you don't accumulate ego, then that total effort will become a surrender in itself. If you accumulate ego, then there is a way: surrender to God.

*In God the seed is developed to its highest extent.*

You are the seed, and God is the manifestation. You are the seed and God is the actuality. You are the potential; he is the actual. God is your destiny, and you are carrying your destiny for many lives without looking at it, because your eyes are fixed somewhere in the future. They don't look to the present. Herenow, everything is as it should be if you are ready to look. Nothing is needed; no doing is needed. Existence is perfect every single moment. It has never been imperfect; it cannot be. If it were imperfect, then how it will become perfect? Who will make it perfect then?

Existence is perfect; nothing at all is needed to be done. If you understand this then surrender is enough. No effort, no *pranayama*, no *bhastrika*, no *shirshasana*, no yoga postures, no meditation, nothing, if you understand this—that existence is perfect as it is. Look in, look out: everything is so perfect that nothing can be done except celebration. A man who surrenders starts celebrating.

# Finding

# The

# Ever

# Present

# Flower

The first question:

*Please explain how a seed can flower without the bit in between.*

HE SEED CAN FLOWER without the gap, without the time gap in between, because the seed is already flowering. You are already that which you can become. If it was not so, then the seed cannot flower right now.

Then time would be needed. Then Zen is not possible. Then only Patanjali is the way. If you are to become something, a time process will be a must. But this is the point to understand: all those who have known, they have also known that becoming is a dream. You are already the being; you are perfect as you are.

Imperfection appears because you are fast asleep. The flower is already flowering; only your eyes are closed. If the seed has to reach to the flower, then much time will be needed, and this is no ordinary flower: God has to flower in you. Then even eternity will not be enough, then it is almost impossible. If you have to flower, then it is almost impossible. It is not going to happen; it cannot happen. Eternity will be needed.

No, that is not the thing. It can happen right now, this very moment! Not even a single moment has to be lost. The question is not of seed becoming a flower. The question is of opening the eyes. You can open your eyes right now, and then you find the flower has always been flowering. It was never otherwise; it could not have been otherwise.

God is always there within you; just a look, and it is manifested. Not that it was hidden in a seed; you were not looking at it. So only this much is needed—that you look at it. Whatsoever you are, look at it, become aware of it. Don't move like a sleepwalker.

That's why it is related that many Zen Masters, when they became awakened, they roared with laughter. Their disciples couldn't understand, their fellow travelers couldn't understand, what happened. Why they are roaring madly? Why this laughter? They were laughing because of the whole absurdity. They were seeking that which was already achieved; they were running after something which was already there within them; they were seeking something somewhere else which was hidden in the seeker himself.

The seeker is the sought; the traveler is the goal. You are not to reach somewhere else. You are to reach only to yourself. This can happen in a single moment; even a fraction of a moment is enough. If the seed has to become a flower, then eternity is not enough because it is a flower of God. If you are already the God, then just a look back, just a look within, then it can happen.

Then why Patanjali? Patanjali is needed because of you. You take such a long time to get out of your sleep, you take such a long time to get out of your dreams, you are so much involved in the dreams, you have so much invested in your dreams, that is why time is needed. Time is not needed because the seed has to become a flower; time is needed because you cannot open your eyes. With closed eyes you have become so much accustomed, it has become a deep habit. Not only that: you have completely forgotten that you are living with closed eyes. You have completely forgotten it! You think that, "What nonsense you are talking. My eyes are already open." And your eyes are closed!

If I say, "Get out of your dreams," you say, "I am already awake," and this too is a dream. You can dream that you are awake; you can dream that your eyes are open. Then much time will be needed—not that the flower was not already flowering—but it was so difficult for you to awake. There are many investments. Those investments have to be understood. The ego is the basic involvement. If you open your eyes, you disappear. Opening the eyes looks like death. It is. So you talk about it, you listen about it, you think about it, but you never open the eyes because if you really open the eyes you also know that you will disappear. Then who will be you? A nobody! A nothingness! This nothingness is there if you open the eyes, so it is better to believe that the eyes are already open, and you remain somebody.

The ego is the first involvement. The ego can exist only while you are asleep, just like dreams can exist only while you are asleep. The ego can exist only while you are asleep—metaphysically asleep, existentially asleep. Open the eyes! First you disappear; then God appears: this is the problem. And you are afraid that you may disappear, but that is the door, so you listen about it, you think about it, but you go on postponing —tomorrow, tomorrow and tomorrow.

That's why Patanjali is needed. Patanjali says no need to open the eyes immediately; there are many steps. You can come out of your sleep in steps, in degrees. Certain things you do today, certain tomorrow, then day after tomorrow, and it is going to take a long time. Patanjali appeals because he gives you time to sleep. He says no need to come out of your sleep right

now; just a turning over will do. Then have a little more
sleep; then do something else. Then by and by, in
degrees. . .

He is a great persuader. He persuades you out of
your sleep. Zen shocks you out of your sleep. That's
why a Zen Master can hit you on your head; never a
Patanjali. A Zen Master can throw you out of the win-
dow; never a Patanjali. Because a Zen Master uses
shock treatment — you can be shocked out of a sleep, so
why go on trying and persuading you? Why waste time?

Patanjali brings you by and by, by and by. He brings
you out and you are not even aware what he is doing.
He is just like a mother. He does just the opposite, but
just like the mother. A mother persuades a child into
sleep. She may sing a lullaby, let the child feel she is
there, no need to be afraid. Repeating the same line
again and again, the child feels seduced into sleep. He
falls into sleep holding the hand of the mother. No need
to be worried. The mother is there and she is singing,
and singing is beautiful. And the mother is not saying
that, "Go into sleep," because that will disturb. She is
simply persuading indirectly. And then by and by she
will take her hand out, and she will cover the blanket
and move from the room, and the child is fast asleep.

Just the same Patanjali does in the reverse order. By
and by he brings you out of your sleep. That's why time
is needed; otherwise the flower is already flowering.
Look! It is already there. Open the eyes and it is there;
open the door and he is standing there waiting for you.
He has been always standing there.

It depends on you. If you like a shock treatment, then
Zen is the path. If you like a very gradual process, then
yoga is the path. Choose! In choosing also you are very
deceptive. You say to me, "How I can choose?" That too
is a trick. Everything is plain. If you need time, choose
Patanjali. If you are afraid of shocks, choose Patanjali.
But choose! Otherwise non-choosing will become the

postponement. Then you say, "It is difficult to choose, and unless I choose how I can move?"

A shock treatment is immediate. It brings you down to the earth immediately. My own methods are shock treatment. They are not gradual. With me you can hope to attain in this life; with Patanjali many lives will be needed. With me you can hope to attain right now also, but you have many things to do before you attain.

You know ego will disappear, you know sex will disappear. There is no possibility of sex, once you attain; it becomes absurd, silly. So you think, "A little more. What is wrong in waiting? Let me enjoy a little more." Anger will not be possible, violence will not be possible, jealousy will not be there; possessiveness, manipulating, they all will disappear.

You suddenly feel, "If all these disappear, then what I will be?"—because you are nothing but a combination of all these, a bundle of all these and if all these disappear, then only nothingness is left. That nothingness scares you. It looks like an abyss. You would like to close your eyes and dream a little more, just as in the morning you are awake but you would like to turn the side just for five minutes and have a little dream more—it was so beautiful.

One night Mulla Nasruddin woke up his wife and told her, "Bring my specs immediately. I was having such a beautiful dream, and more is promised."

And desires go on promising you—more is always promised—and they say, "Do this and that, and why be in a hurry when enlightenment is always possible? You can attain any time; there is no hurry. You can postpone it. It is a question of eternity, a concern of eternity; why not enjoy this moment?"

You are not enjoying but the mind says, "Why not enjoy this moment?" And you have never enjoyed; because a man without inner understanding cannot enjoy anything. He simply suffers; everything becomes a suffering to him. Love—a thing like love—he suffers even that. The most beautiful phenomenon possible to a man asleep is love, but he suffers even through that. Nothing better is possible when you are asleep. Love is the greatest possibility, but even you suffer from that. Because it is not a question of love or something else— sleep is suffering, so whatsoever happens you will suffer. Sleep turns every dream into a nightmare. It starts beautifully, but something somewhere goes always wrong. In the end you reach to hell.

Every desire leads to hell. They say every road leads to Rome—I don't know, but of one thing I am certain: every desire leads to hell. In the beginning desire gives you much hope, dreams: that is the trick. That's how you are trapped. If the desire from the very beginning says, "Be alert: I am leading you to hell," you won't follow it. The desire promises you the heaven, and promises you—"Just a few steps and you will reach it; just come with me"—allures you, hypnotizes you and promises you many things, and you, being in suffering, think, "What is wrong in trying? Let us try a little this desire also."

That too will lead you to the hell because desire as such is a path to hell. Hence, Buddha says, "Unless you become desireless, you cannot be blissful." Desire is suffering, desire is a dream, and desire exists only when you are asleep. When you are awake and alert, desires cannot befool you. Then you see through; then everything is so clear that you cannot be befooled. How money can befool you and say that you will be very, very happy when there is money? Then look to rich people: they are in hell also—maybe a rich hell, but it makes no difference. A richer hell is going to be worse than a poor hell. Now they have attained money, and they are simply in a state of constant nervousness.

Mulla Nasruddin accumulated much wealth, and then he entered a hospital, because he couldn't sleep and he was nervous and constantly trembling and afraid—

afraid of nothing in particular. A poor man is afraid of something in particular; a rich man is simply afraid. If you are afraid about something in particular, something can be done. But he is simply afraid. he does not know why, because he has everything; there is no need to be afraid, but he is simply afraid and trembling.

He was entered into the hospital, and for the breakfast few things were brought, and in those few things was a bowl of quivering gelatin. He said, "No. I cannot eat this." The doctor asked, "Why you are so adamant about it?" He said, "I cannot eat anything more nervous than me!"

But a rich man is nervous. What is his nervousness, the fear? Why he is so scared? Because every desire fulfilled, and still the frustration remains. Now he cannot even dream, because all dreams he has passed through; they lead nowhere. He cannot dream and he cannot gather courage to open the eyes also, because there are involvements. He has promised many things in his sleep.

When Buddha disappeared one night from his palace, he wanted to tell his wife that, "I am going." He wanted to touch the child who was just a day before born, because he would not be back again. He went to the very door of the room. He looked at the wife. She was so fast asleep, must have been dreaming; her face was beautiful, smiling, child in her arms. Then he waited for few seconds on the door; then he turned. He wanted to say, but then he became afraid. If he said something, then the wife is bound to cry and weep and create a scene.

And he is afraid of himself also, because if she weeps and cries, then he may become aware of his own promises, that "I will love you forever and ever, and I will be with you forever and ever." And what about this child who is only one day born? And she will, of course, bring the child before me, and she will say, "Look what you have done to me. Then why you gave birth to this child? And now who will be his father? And am I alone responsible for him? And you are escaping like a coward." All these thoughts came to him, because in sleep everybody promises. Everybody goes on giving promises not knowing how he can fulfill them, but in sleep it happens because nobody is conscious what is happening.

Suddenly he became aware that these things will be brought and then the family will gather—and the father and everybody else—and he is the only son of the father, and the father is looking at him, and in his sleep he has promised him also. Then he simply escaped: he simply escaped like a thief.

After twelve years, when he came back, the wife asked him the first thing that had come to his mind that night when he was leaving. The wife asked, "Why didn't you tell me? The first thing I would like to ask—for these twelve years I was waiting for you—why didn't you tell me? What type of love is this? You simply left me. You are a coward."

And Buddha listened silently. And the wife was silent and he said, "These all thoughts had come to me. I had come just to the door, I had even opened the door. I looked at you; in sleep I had promised many things. But if I am going to be awake, if I am getting out of the sleep, then I cannot keep the promises given in sleep. And if I try to keep the promises, then I cannot awake.

"So you are right. You may think I am a coward; you may think that I escaped from the palace like a thief, not like a warrior, not like a man of courage. But I tell you, exactly opposite is the case, because when I was escaping, to me at that moment, that was the moment of greatest bravery because my whole being was saying, 'This is not good. Don't be a coward.' And if I had stopped, if I had listened to my sleepy being, then there was no possibility for me to awake.

"And now I come to you; now I can fulfill something,

because only a man who is enlightened can fulfill. A man who is ignorant, how he can fulfill anything? Now I come to you. That moment if I had stopped I couldn't give you anything, but now I bring a great treasure with me, and now I can give it to you. Don't weep, don't cry; open the eyes and look at me. I am not the same man who had left that night. A totally different being has come to your door. I am not your husband. You may be my wife, because that is your attitude. Look at me — I am totally a different person. Now I bring treasures for you. I can make you also aware and enlightened."

The wife listened. The same problem always came to everybody. She started thinking about the child. If she becomes a sannyasin and moves with this beggar — her ex-husband, now he is a beggar — if she moves. . .and what will happen to the child? She has not said anything, but Buddha said, "I know what you are thinking, because I have passed that period where promises given in the sleepy state all crowd together and say, 'What are you doing? — your child. . .' You are thinking that, 'Let the child become a little more aged, let him be married, then he can take over the palace and the kingdom,' and then you will follow. But remember, there is no future, no tomorrow. Either you follow me right now or you don't follow me."

But the wife. . . And a feminine mind is more asleep than a male mind. There are reasons for it, because a woman is a greater dreamer, she lives more in hopes and dreams. She has to be a greater sleeper, otherwise it will be difficult for nature to use her as the mother. A woman must be in deep hypnotic state, only then she can carry a child nine months in the womb and suffer, and then give birth and suffer, and then bring up this child and suffer, and then one day this child simply leaves her and goes to another woman. . .and suffer.

It is such a long suffering, a woman is bound to be a greater sleeper than man. Otherwise, how can you suffer so much? And she always hopes. Then she hopes with another child, then with another child, and her whole life is wasted.

So Buddha said, "I know what you are thinking, and I know you are a greater dreamer than me. But now I have come to cut all the roots of your sleep. Bring the child. Where is my son? Bring him." The feminine mind played a trick again. She brought Rahul, the child who was twelve years of age now, and she said, "This is your father. Look at him — he has become a beggar — and ask him what is your heritage, what he can give to you. This is your father; he is a coward! He escaped like a thief not even telling me, and he left a one-day-old child. Ask him your heritage!"

Buddha laughed, and he told Ananda, "Bring my begging bowl." And he gave the begging bowl to Rahul, and he said, "This is my heritage. I make you a beggar. You are initiated. You become a sannyasin." And he said to his wife, "I cut the very root. Now there is no need to dream. You also awake because this was the root. Rahul is already a sannyasin; you also awake. Yashodhara, you also awake, and become a sannyasin."

The moment always comes when you are in the transit period from where sleep turns into awakening. The whole past will hold you back, and past is powerful. Future is powerless for a sleepy man. For a man who is not sleepy, future is powerful; for a man who is fast asleep, past is powerful, because a man who is fast asleep knows only dreams that he had dreamed in the past. He is not aware of any future. Even if he thinks about future, it is nothing but past reflected again; it is just past projected again. Only a man who is aware becomes aware of the future. Then past is nothing.

Keep it in the mind. You may not be able to understand right now, but some day you may understand. For a sleepy man, cause is more powerful than the effect; seed is more powerful than the flower. For a man who is awake, effect is more powerful than the cause, flower is more powerful than the seed. The logic of sleep is: the cause produces the effect, seed produces the flower. The logic of awakening is just the reverse: it is flower who produces the seed; it is effect who produces the cause; it is future who produces the past, not the past that produces the future. But for a sleepy mind, the past, the dead, the gone, is more powerful. It is not. . .

The yet-to-be is more powerful: the yet-to-be-born is more powerful because life is there. Past has no life. How it can be powerful? Past is already graveyard. Life has already moved from there: that's why it is past. Life has left it, but graveyards are very powerful for you. The yet-to-be, the yet-to-be-born, the fresh, that which is going to happen, for a man of awakening that becomes more powerful. The past cannot hold him back.

The past holds you back. You always think about past commitments; you always linger around the graveyard. You go again and again to visit the graveyard and pay your respects to the dead. Always pay respects to the yet-to-be-born, because life is there.

*Please explain how a seed can flower without the bit in between.*

Yes, it can flower because it is already flowering. It creates the seed, not the seed the flower. It is flower that is going to be, has created the whole seed. But for you to remember is: only an opening is needed. Open the doors; the sun is there waiting for you. Life is not, in fact, a progress in reality. It appears like progress in sleep.

The being is already there—everything as it is already, perfect, absolute, ecstatic—nothing can be added, there is no way to improve upon it. Then what is needed? Only one thing, that you become conscious and see it. This can happen in two ways. Either you can be shocked out of your sleep: that is Zen. Or, you can be brought, persuaded, out of your sleep: that is yoga. Choose! Just don't hang in between.

The second question:

*Is surrender to Ishwara — God — and surrender to the guru the same?*

Surrender doesn't depend on the object. It is a quality that you bring in your being. To whom you surrender is irrelevant. Any object will do. You can surrender to a tree; you can surrender to a river; you can surrender to anything — to your wife, to your husband, to your child. The problem is not there in the object; any object will do. The problem is to surrender.

The happening happens because of surrendering, not because to whom you have surrendered. And this is the most beautiful thing to understand: whomsoever you surrender, that object becomes the God. There is no question of surrendering to God. Where will you find God to surrender? You will never find. Surrender! And to whomsoever you surrender, the God is there. The child becomes the God, the husband becomes the God, the wife becomes the God, the guru becomes the God, even a stone can become God.

Even through stones people have attained, because it is not a question at all to what you surrender. You surrender, and that brings the whole thing, that opens the door. Surrendering, the effort to surrender, brings an opening to you. And if you are open to a stone you become open to the whole existence, because it is only a question of opening. How can you be open to a stone and not open to the tree? Once you know the opening, once you enjoy the euphoria that it brings, the ecstasy that happens just by opening to a stone, then you cannot find such a foolish man who will close immediately to the remaining existence. When even opening to a stone gives such ecstatic experience, then why not open to all?

In the beginning one surrenders to something, and then one is surrendered to all. That is the meaning that if you surrender to a Master, in the experience of surrendering, you have learned a clue; now you can surrender to all. The Master becomes just a passage to be passed through. He becomes a door, and through that door you can look at the whole sky. Remember, you cannot find God to surrender, but many people think that way; they are very tricky people. They think, "When God is there, we will surrender." Now this is impossible because God is there only if you surrender. Surrender makes anything God. Surrender gives you the eyes, and everything that is brought to these eyes becomes divine. Divinity, divineness, is a quality given by surrendering.

In India, Christians, Jews and Mohammedans laugh about Hindus, because they may be worshipping a tree or they may be worshipping a stone—not even carved, not even a statue. They can find a stone by the side of the road, and they can make a god out of it immediately. No artist is needed because surrender is the art. No carving, not a valuable stone is needed, not even marble. Any ordinary stone, discarded—it cannot be sold in the market and that's why it is lying there by the side of the road—and Hindus can make immediately a god out of it. If you can surrender, it becomes divine. The eyes of surrender cannot find anything else than the divine.

Others have laughed; they couldn't understand. They think that these people are stone worshippers, idol worshippers. They are not! Hindus have been misunderstood. They are not idol worshippers. They have found a key, and that key is that you can make anything divine if you surrender. And if you don't surrender then you can go on searching for God for millions of lives. You will never meet him, because you don't have the quality which meets, which can meet, which can find. So the question is of a subjective surrender, not of the object to whom to surrender.

But, of course, there are problems. You cannot so

suddenly surrender to a stone because your mind goes on saying, "This is just a stone. What are you doing?" And if the mind goes on saying, "This is a stone; what are you doing?"—then you cannot surrender, because surrender needs your totality.

Hence, the significance of a Master. A Master means somebody who is standing on the boundary—boundary of the human and the divine. One who has been a human being like you, but is no more like you—something else has happened—who is a plus, a human being plus. So if you look to his past, he is just like you—but if you look to his present and the future, then you look to the plus. Then he is the divine.

It is difficult to surrender to a stone, to a river—very, very difficult—even to surrender to a Master is so difficult. Then surrendering to a stone is bound to be very difficult, because whenever you see a Master, then again your mind said that this is a human being like you, so why surrender to him? And your mind cannot see the present; the mind can see only the past—that this man is born like you, eats, sleeps like you, so why surrender to him? He is just like you.

He is, and yet he is not. He is both Jesus and Christ —Jesus the man, the son of man, and Christ, the plus point. If you watch only the visible, then he is the stone; you cannot surrender. If you love, if you become intimate, if you allow his presence to go deep in you, if you can find a rapport—that is the word; rapport with his being—then suddenly you become aware of the plus. He is more than human. In some unknown way, he has something that you have not got. In some invisible way, he has penetrated beyond the boundary of the human. But this you can feel only if there is a rapport.

That is what Patanjali says, *shraddha*—trust; trust creates rapport. Rapport is an inner harmony of the two invisibles; love is a rapport. With somebody you simply fit as if you both were born for each other. You call it love. In a moment, even at the first sight, somebody simply fits with you, as if you were created together and were separated; now you have met again.

In the old mythologies all over the world, it is said that man and woman were created together. In Indian mythology they have a very beautiful myth. The myth is that a wife and husband were created in the very beginning as twins, brother and sister. Together they were born — wife and husband as twins, fitting together in one womb. There was a rapport from the very beginning. From the first moment there was a rapport. They were together in the womb holding each other, and that is rapport. Then, due to some misfortune, that phenomenon disappeared from the earth.

But the myth says that still there is a relationship. A man and a woman. . . The man may be born here and the woman may be born somewhere in Africa, in America, but there is a rapport, and unless they find each other there will be difficulty. And it is very difficult to find each other. The world is so vast, and you don't know where to seek and where to find. If it happens, it happens by accident.

Now scientists also believe that sooner or later we will be able to judge the rapport by scientific instruments, and before somebody goes for marriage, the couple has to go to a lab so that they can find whether their bio-energy fits or not. If it is not fitting, then they are in an illusion. This marriage cannot. . . They may be thinking that they will be very happy, but they cannot be because the inner bio-energy does not fit.

So you may like the nose of the woman and the woman may like your eyes, but that is not the point. Liking the eyes won't help, liking the nose won't help, because after two days nobody looks at the nose and nobody looks at the eyes. Then the problem is of bio-energy. The inner energies meeting and mixing with each other; otherwise they will repel. It is just like if you transfuse blood; either your body accepts it or rejects it, because there are types of blood. If it is the same type, only then the body accepts it; otherwise it simply rejects.

The same happens in a marriage. If the bio-energy accepts, it accepts, and there is no conscious way to know about it. Love is very fallacious, because love is always focused on something. The voice of the woman is good, and you are allured. But that is not the point. It is a partial thing. The whole must fit. Your bio-energies should accept each other so totally that deep down you become a one person. This is rapport. It happens in love rarely because how to find? — it is still difficult. Just falling in love is not a sure criterion. Out of one thousand, nine hundred ninety-nine times it fails. Love has proved a failure.

Even a greater rapport happened with a Master. It is greater than love. It is *shraddha* — trust. Not only your bio-energy meets and fits, but your very soul fits together. That's why, whenever somebody becomes a disciple, the whole world thinks he is mad; because the whole world cannot see what is the point. Why are you going mad after this man? And you cannot explain it also, because it cannot be explained. You may be even not aware consciously what has happened, but with a man, suddenly, you are in trust. Suddenly something meets, becomes one. That is rapport.

It is difficult to have that rapport with a stone. Because it is even difficult to have that rapport with a living Master, how can you have it with a stone? But if it happens, immediately the Master becomes a God. For the disciple, the Master is always a God. He may not be a God for others; that is not the point. But for a disciple he is the God, and through him the doors of divineness open. Then you have the key — that this inner rapport is the key, this surrender. Then you can try it: surrender to a river. . .

You must have read Hermann Hesse's "Siddhartha".

He learns many things from the river. You cannot learn from a Buddha, just watching the river, so many moods of the river. He has become a ferryboat man just watching thousands of climates around it. Sometimes the river is happy and dancing, and sometimes very, very sad, as if not moving at all — sometimes very angry and roaring, against the whole existence, and sometimes so calm and peaceful like a Buddha. And Siddhartha simply a ferryman — passing the river, living near the river, watching the river, with nothing else to do. It becomes a deep meditation and a rapport, and through the river and the "riverness" of it he attains: he attains to the same glimpse as Heraclitus.

You can step in the same river and you cannot. The river is the same and not the same. It is a flow, and through the river and the rapport with it he comes to know the whole existence as a river — a "riverness".

It can happen with anything. The basic to remember is surrendering.

*Is surrender to* Ishwara — *God — and surrender to a guru the same?*

Yes! Surrender is always the same. It is just up to you to whom you can be able to surrender. Find the man, seek the river, and surrender. It is a risk — the greatest risk possible. That's why it is so difficult to surrender. It is a risk! You are moving in the unknown territory and you are giving so much power to a man or to something you surrender.

If you surrender to me you are giving total power to me. Then my yes is your yes, then my no is your no. Even in the day I say it is night, you say, "Yes, it is night." You are giving total power to somebody. The ego resists. The mind says, "This is not good. Keep the control yourself. Who knows where this man will lead you? Who knows, he may say, 'Jump from the hilltop,' and then you will be dead. Who knows, this man may manipulate you, control you, exploit you." The mind will bring all these things. It is a risk, and the mind is taking all the security measures.

The mind is saying, "Be watchful. Watch this man a little more." If you listen to the mind, surrender is not possible. Mind is right! It is a risk! But whenever you take, it is going to be a risk. Watching won't help much. You can watch forever, and may not be able to decide because the mind can never decide. Mind is confusion. It is never decisive. You have to bypass mind someday or other, and you have to tell the mind, "You wait. I go: I will take the jump and see what happens."

What you have got to lose really? I'm always wondering what you have got that you are so afraid to lose, what exactly that you are bringing when you surrender. You have nothing. You can gain out of it, but you cannot lose because you have nothing. You can always be profited out of it, but there is no possibility of any loss because you do not have anything to lose.

You must have heard Karl Marx's famous maxim, "Proletarians of the world unite because you have nothing to lose but your chains." That may be true, may not be true. But for a seeker this is exactly the thing. What you have got to lose except your chains, your ignorance, your misery? But people become very much attached to their misery also — to their very misery they cling as if it is a treasure. If you want to take their misery away, they create all sorts of barriers.

I have been watching these barriers and these tricks with thousands of people. Even if you want to take their misery, they cling. They indicate a certain thing because they don't have anything else, this is the only treasure that they have. Don't take it away because it is always better to have something than nothing. That is their logic: it is always better to have something — at least this misery is there — than nothing, than to be completely empty, than to be nobody.

Even if you are miserable, you are somebody. Even if

you have a hell within you, at least you have something. But watch this, observe this, and when you surrender remember you have nothing else to give. A Master is taking your misery, nothing else. He is not taking your life because you don't have. He is taking only your death. He is not taking anything valuable from you because you don't have it. He is taking only the rubbish, the junkyard that you have collected through many lives, and you are sitting on the heap of the junkyard and you think this is your kingdom.

He is not taking anything. If you are ready to give your misery to him, you will become capable to receive his bliss. This is the surrender, and then the Master becomes a god. Anything, anybody you surrender becomes divine. Surrender makes divineness, surrender creates divineness. Surrender is a creative force.

The third question:

*Is a Master needed after* satori?

Yes! Even more so, because *satori* is just a glimpse, and a glimpse is dangerous because now you enter the territory of the unknown. Before it, Master is not necessary. Before it you were moving in the known world. Only after *satori* he becomes absolutely necessary, because now somebody is needed to hold your hand and to lead you towards that which is not simply a glimpse, but becomes an absolute reality. After *satori* you have the taste, and the taste creates more desire. And the taste becomes so magnetic that you would like to rush into it madly. Now the Master is needed.

After *satori*, many more things are going to happen. *Satori* is like seeing the peak of Gourishankar, Everest, from the plains. Some day, a clear morning, a sunny morning, and mist is not there, you can see from thousands of miles away the beautiful peak of Gourishankar rising high in the sky. This is *satori*. Now the actual traveling starts. Now the whole world looks useless.

This is a turning point. Now all that you knew becomes useless, all that you had becomes a burden. Now the world, the life that you had lived up to now, simply disappears like a dream because the greater has happened. And this is *satori*, a glimpse. Soon the mist will be there, and the peak will not be visible. The clouds will come and the peak will disappear. Now you will be in an absolute uncertain state of consciousness.

The first thing will be whether whatsoever you have seen was real or just a dream, because where it is now? It has disappeared. It was just a breakthrough, just a gap, and you are back—thrown to your own world.

Suspicions will arise: whatsoever you have seen, was it true? Was it really there or you dreamed about it or you imagined it? And there are possibilities. Many people imagine, so the suspicion is not wrong. Many times you will imagine, and you cannot make the distinction, what is real and what is unreal. Only a Master can say that, "Yes, don't be worried. It was real," or a Master can say, "Drop, throw it! It was just imaginary."

Only one who has known the peak—not from the plains—only one who has attained to the peak, only one who has become the peak himself, only he can tell you because he has the criterion, he has the touchstone. He can say, "Throw it! Rubbish! It is just your imagination," because when seekers go on thinking about these things, the mind starts dreaming.

Many people come to me. Only one percent of them have the real thing; ninety-nine percent bring unreal things. But it is difficult for them to decide—impossible, not difficult—they cannot decide. You suddenly feel an upsurge of energy in your backbone, in the spine: how you will decide whether it is real or unreal? You have been thinking too much about it; you have been desiring also. Unconsciously you are sowing seeds that it should happen, the kundalini should rise. Then you have been reading Patanjali, then you have been talking about it, then you meet people who say their kundalini has risen. Your ego, and then everything mixed. . .

Suddenly one day, you feel the upsurge; it is nothing but a creation of the mind—just to satisfy you—that, "Don't be worried: don't be so much worried. Look! Your kundalini has arisen," and just mind imagining. Then who will decide? And how you will decide?— because you don't know the true. Only truth can become the criterion to decide whether this is true or untrue.

A Master is needed even more after first *satori*. There are three *satoris*. The first *satori* is just a glimpse. This is possible even sometimes through drugs; this is possible through many other things—sometimes accidents. Sometimes you were climbing a tree and you fell down, and it was such a shock that the mind stopped for a single moment, and the glimpse will be there, and you will feel so euphoric that you are taken out of your body, you have known something.

Within a second you are back, the mind starts functioning: it was simply a shock. Through electric shock it is possible, through insulin shock it is possible, through drugs it is possible. Even sometimes in illness it happens. You are so weak that the mind cannot function; suddenly you have a glimpse. Through sex it is possible. In the orgasm, when the whole body vibrates, it is possible.

The first glimpse is not necessarily through religious effort. That's why LSD, mescaline, marijuana, have become so much important and appealing. The first glimpse is possible, and you can be caught because of the first glimpse in a drug. It can become a permanent trip; then it is very dangerous because glimpses won't help. They can help, but there is not necessarily help coming from them. They can help only around a Master, because then he will say, "Now don't be after the glimpse. You have got the glimpse, now start traveling to reach the peak." Because it is not only to reach the peak; finally one has to become the peak.

These are the three stages: first is glimpse — this is possible through many ways, not necessarily religious. Even an atheist can have the glimpse, a person who is not interested in religion can have the glimpse. Drugs, chemicals can give you the glimpse. Even after an operation, when you are coming out of chloroform, you can have the glimpse. While the chloroform is given to you and you are going deeper and deeper, you can have the glimpse.

Many people have attained to first *satori;* that is not very, very significant. It can be used as a step for the second *satori.* Second *satori* is to reach the peak. That never happens accidentally. That happens only through methods, techniques, schools, because it is a long effort to reach the second *satori.*

And then there is the third *satori,* what Patanjali calls *samadhi:* that third is to become the peak. Because from the second also you can come down. You reach to the peak; it may be unbearable. Bliss is also sometimes unbearable — not only pain, bliss also — it is too much; one comes back to the plains.

To live on a high peak is difficult — very difficult! — and one would like to come back. Unless you become the peak itself, unless the experiencer becomes the experience, it can be lost. And up to the third — *samadhi* — a Master is needed. Only when the final *samadhi,* the ultimate, has happened, a Master is not needed.

The last question:

*While listening to you, many times certain words go very deep, and there is a sudden clarity and understanding. This seems to happen only when I am attending to the words spoken*

*by you. But, the peace that descends while*
*listening to you without any particular attention*
*to your words is equally blissful, but then the*
*words and their meaning get lost. Please give a*
*guide to the art of listening to you, as it is one*
*of your best meditations.*

Don't be much bothered by words and the meaning. If
you pay much attention to the words and the meaning,
it becomes an intellectual thing. Of course, sometimes
you will attain to clarity. Suddenly the clouds disappear
and the sun is there, but these will be only momentary
things and this clarity will not help much; next moment
it is gone. Intellectual clarity is not of much use.

If you listen to the words and their meaning you may
understand many things, but you will not understand
me and you will not understand yourself also. Those
many things are not worth. You don't bother about
words and meanings; you listen to me as if I am not a
speaker but a singer, as if I am not talking to you in
words, but talking to you in sounds, as if I am a poet!

No need to try the meaning, what I mean. Just listening to me without paying any attention to words and
meanings, a different quality of clarity will come to
you. You will feel blissful: that's the real clarity. You
will feel happy; you will feel peaceful and silent and
calm. That is the real meaning.

Because I am here not to explain certain things to
you, but to create a certain quality within your being. I
am talking not to explain: my talking is a creative phenomenon. I am not trying to explain to you something
— that you can do through books and there are millions
of other ways to understand these things — I am here to
transform you.

Listen to me — simply, innocently, without creating
any worry about words and their meanings. Drop that
clarity; that is not of much use. When you simply listen
to me, transparent, the intellect no more there — heart to

heart, depth to depth, being to being — then the speaker disappears and the listener also. Then I am not here and you are also not here. A rapport exists; the listener and the speaker have become one. In that oneness, you will be transformed. To attain to that oneness is the meditation. Make it a meditation, not a contemplation, not a reflection. Then something greater than words is communicated — something beyond meanings. The real meaning, the ultimate meaning, is transferred — something that is not in the scriptures and cannot be.

You can read Patanjali yourself. A little effort and you will understand him. I am not talking here so that you become capable of understanding Patanjali; no, that is not the point at all. Patanjali is just an excuse, a peg. I am hanging something that is beyond scriptures on him.

If you listen to my words, you will understand Patanjali, there will be a clarity. But if you listen to my sound, if you listen not to the words but to me, then the real meaning will be revealed to you, and that meaning has nothing to do with Patanjali. That meaning is a transmission beyond scriptures.

# The
# Master
# Of
# Masters

*Being beyond the limits of time he is the Master of Masters.*

*He is known as AUM.*

*Repeat and meditate on AUM.*

*Repeating and meditating on AUM brings about the disappearance of all obstacles and an awakening of a new consciousness.*

**P**ATANJALI IS TALKING about the phenomenon of God. God is not the creator. For Patanjali, God is the ultimate flowering of individual consciousness. Everybody is on the way to become a god. Not only you, but the stones, the rocks, every unit of existence is on the way to become a god. Some have become already; some are becoming; some will become.

God is not the creator, but the culmination, the peak, the ultimate of existence. He is not in the beginning: he is in the end. And, of course, in a sense, he is in the beginning also, because in the end only that can flower which has always been from the very beginning as a seed. God is the potentiality, the hidden possibility: this has to be remembered. So Patanjali has not a single God, he has infinite gods. The whole existence is full of gods.

Once you understand Patanjali's conception of God, then God is not to be really worshipped. You have to become one; that is the only worship. If you go on worshipping God, that won't help. In fact, that is foolish. The worship, real worship, should consist in becoming yourself a god. The whole effort should be to bring your potentiality to the point where it explodes into an actuality—where the seed is broken and that which was hidden from eternity becomes manifested. You are God unmanifested, and the effort is how to bring the unmanifested to the manifested level—how to bring it to the plane of manifestation.

*Being beyond the limits of time, he is the Master of Masters.*

He is talking about his conception of God. When somebody becomes a flower, when somebody becomes a lotus of being, many things happen to him and many things start happening through him into existence. He becomes a great power, an infinite power, and through him, in many ways, others are helped to become gods in their own right.

*Being beyond the limits of time, he is the Master of Masters.*

There are three types of Masters. One is not exactly a Master; rather a teacher. A teacher is one who teaches, who helps people to know about things, without himself realizing them. Sometimes teachers can attract thousands of people. The only thing needed is they should be good teachers. They may not have known themselves, but they can talk, they can argue, they can preach, and many people can get attracted through their talks, their preaching, their sermons. And talking continuously about God, they may be befooling themselves. By and by they may start feeling that they know.

When you talk about a thing, the greatest danger is that you may start believing that you know. In the beginning when you start to talk, to teach — and teaching has some appeal because it is very ego-fulfilling — when somebody listens to you attentively, deep down it fulfills your ego that you know and he doesn't know. You are the knower and he is ignorant.

It happened: a priest, a great priest, was called into a madhouse to say a few words to the inmates of that house. The priest was not expecting much, but he was surprised. One madman listened to him so attentively, that he had never seen any man listen to him so attentively. He was just bending forward; each word he was taking into his heart. The man was not even blinking. He was so attentive — as if hypnotized.

When the priest has finished his sermon, he saw that the same man reached to the superintendent and said something to him. He was curious. As soon as possible, he asked the superintendent, "What that man was saying to you? Was he saying something about my sermon?" The superintendent said, "Yes." Asked the priest, "Would you mind to tell me what he said?" The superintendent was a little bit reluctant, but then he said, "Yes. The man said, 'See? I am in and he is out!' "

A teacher is exactly in the same place, in the same boat, as you are. He is also an inmate. He has nothing more than you — just a little more information. Information means nothing. You can accumulate; ordinary, average intelligence is needed to accumulate information. One need not be a genius, one need not be very talented. Just average intelligence is enough. You can accumulate information. You can go on accumulating; you can become a teacher.

A teacher is one who knows without knowing. He attracts people, if he is a good talker, a good writer, if he has a personality, if he has a certain charisma about him, magnetic eyes, a forceful body. And by and by he becomes more and more skillful. But the people around him cannot be disciples, they will remain students. Even if he pretends that he is a Master, he cannot make you a disciple. At the most he can make you a student. A student is one who is in search of more information and a teacher is one who has accumulated more information. This is the first type of master—who is not a Master at all.

Then there is a second type of Master—who has known himself. Whatsoever he says, he can say like Heraclitus: "I have searched." Or like Buddha he can say, "I have found." Heraclitus is more polite. He was talking to people who could not have understood if he had said like Buddha, "I have found." Buddha says, "I am the most perfect enlightened man that has ever happened." It looks egoistic, but it is not and he was talking to his disciples who could have understood that there was no ego at all.

Heraclitus was talking to people who were not disciples—just ordinary people. They will not have understood. Politely he says, "I have searched," and leaves the other part—that, "I have found" for your imagination. Buddha never says, "I have searched." He says, "I have found! And this enlightenment has never happened before. It is utterly absolute."

One who has found is a Master. He will accept disciples. Students are prohibited; students cannot go there by themselves. Even if they drift and reach somehow, they will leave as soon as possible because he will not be helping you to gather more knowledge. He will try to transform you. He will give you being, not knowledge. He will give you more being, not more knowledge. He will make you centered, and the center is somewhere near the navel, not in the head.

Whosoever lives in the head is eccentric. The word is beautiful: the English word eccentric means off center.

Really, he is mad whosoever lives in the head—head is the periphery. You can live in your feet or you can live in your head: the distance from the center is the same. The center is somewhere near the navel.

A teacher helps you to be more and more head-rooted; a Master will uproot you from the head and replant you. Exactly it is a replanting, so much pain is there—bound to be—suffering, anguish, because when you replant, the plant has to be uprooted from the soil. It has always been. And then, again, it has to be planted in a new soil. It will take time! The old leaves will drop. The whole plant will pass through anguish, uncertainty, not knowing whether he is going to survive or not. It is a rebirth! With a teacher there is no rebirth; with a Master there is a rebirth.

Socrates is right: he says, "I am a midwife." Yes, a Master is a midwife! He helps you to be reborn. But that means you will have to die: only then you can be reborn. So a Master is not only a midwife; Socrates says only the half thing. A Master is a murderer also—a murderer plus a midwife. First he will kill you as you are, and only the new can come out of you then. Out of your death, the resurrection.

A teacher never changes you. Whatsoever you are, whomsoever you are, he simply gives you more information. He adds in you; he retains the continuity. He may modify you, he may refine you. You may become more cultured, more polished. But you will remain the same: the base will be the same.

With a Master, a discontinuity happens. Your past becomes as if it was never yours—as if it belonged to somebody else, as if you dreamed it. It was not real; it was a nightmare. The continuity breaks. There is a gap. The old drops and the new comes, and between these two there is a gap. That gap is the problem; that gap has to be passed. In that gap many simply become scared and go back, run fast and cling to their old past.

A Master helps you to cross this gap, but for a

teacher there is nothing like that; there is no problem. A teacher helps you to learn more; a Master — the first job is to help you to unlearn: that is the difference.

Somebody asked Ramana Maharshi that, "I have come from very far to learn from you. Teach me!" Ramana laughed and said, "If you have come to learn, then go somewhere else because here we do the unlearning. Here we don't teach. You already know too much; that is your problem. More learning and there will be more problems. We teach how to unlearn, how to unwind."

A Master attracts disciples, a teacher — students. What is a disciple? Everything has to be understood minutely; then only you will be able to understand Patanjali. Who is a disciple? What is the difference between a student and a disciple? A student is in search of knowledge, a disciple in search of transformation, mutation. He is fed up with himself. He has come to a point to realize that, "As I am, I am worthless — dust, nothing else. As I am it is of no value."

He has come to attain a new birth, a new being. He is ready to pass through the cross, through the pangs of death and rebirth; hence, the word disciple. The word disciple comes from discipline. He is ready to pass through any discipline. Whatsoever the Master says, he is ready to follow. He has followed his own mind up to now, for many lives, and he has reached nowhere. He has listened to his own mind, and he got more and more into trouble. Now a point has come where he realizes that, "Enough of this!"

He comes and surrenders to the Master. This is the discipline, the first step. He says, "Now I will listen to you. I have listened enough of my own; to my mind I have been a follower, a disciple, and it leads nowhere. I have realized this. Now you are my Master." That means, "Now you are my mind. Whatsoever you say, I will listen. Wherever you lead, I will go. I will not question you because that question will come from my mind."

A disciple is one who has learned one thing through life — that your mind is the troublemaker, your mind is the root cause of your miseries. Your mind always says, "Somebody else is the cause of my miseries, not me." A disciple is one who has learned that this is trick, this is a trap of the mind. It always says, "Somebody else is responsible; I am not responsible." This is how it saves itself, protects, remains secure. A disciple is one who has understood that this is wrong — this is a trick of the mind.

Once you feel this whole absurdity of the mind. . . It leads you into desire: desire leads you into frustration. It leads you into success: every success becomes a failure. It attracts you towards beauty, and every beauty proves ugly. It leads you on and on; it never fulfills any promise. It gives you promises. . . No, not even a single promise is fulfilled. It gives you doubt: doubt becomes a worm in the heart — poisonous. It does not allow you to trust, and without trust there is no growth. When you understand this whole thing, then only you can become a disciple.

When you come to the Master, symbolically you put your head into his feet. This is dropping your head: this is putting your head into his feet. Now you say, "Now I will remain headless. Now, whatsoever you say will be my life." This is the surrender. A Master has disciples who are ready to die and be reborn.

Then there is third — a Master of Masters. A teacher of students first; a Master of disciples second; and then the third, a Master of Masters. Patanjali says when a Master becomes a god — and to become a god means one who transcends time; for whom time does not exist, ceases to exist; for him there is no time; one who has come to understand the timelessness, the eternity; who has not only changed and become good, who has not only changed and become aware, who has gone beyond time—he has become a Master of Masters. Now he is a god!

What will he be doing then, a Master of Masters? This stage comes only when a Master leaves the body— never before it. Because in the body you can be aware, in the body you can realize that there is no time. But body has a biological clock. It feels hunger, and after a time gap again hunger—satiety and hunger, sleep, disease, health. In the night the body has to go to sleep; in the morning it has to wake. Body has a biological clock. So the third Master happens only when a Master leaves the body—when he is not to come back to the body again.

Buddha has two terms. First he calls it *nirvana*, enlightenment, when Buddha became enlightened but remained in the body. That is enlightenment, *nirvana*. Then after forty years he left the body; he calls it the absolute *nirvana—Mahaparinirvana*. Now he becomes a Master of Masters, and he has remained a Master of Masters.

Every Master, when he leaves the body permanently, when he is not to come back again, he becomes a Master of Masters. Mohammed, Jesus, Mahavira, Buddha, Patanjali, they have remained Master of Masters, and they have continuously been guiding—Masters not disciples.

Whenever somebody becomes a Master on the path of Patanjali, immediately there is a contact with Patanjali whose soul floats into the infinite, the individual consciousness, which he calls God. Whenever a person following Patanjali's path becomes a Master, enlightened, immediately there is a communication with the original Master who is now a god.

Whenever somebody following Buddha becomes enlightened, immediately a relationship comes into existence. Suddenly he is joined with Buddha—Buddha who is no more in the body, Buddha who is no more in time and no more in space, but still is — Buddha who has become one with totality, but still is.

This is very paradoxical and very difficult to understand because we cannot understand anything which is beyond time. Our whole understanding is within time; our whole understanding is within space. When somebody says Buddha exists beyond time and space, it makes no sense to us.

When you say Buddha exists beyond space, it means he does not exist anywhere in particular. And how somebody can exist without existing anywhere in particular? He exists, simply exists! You cannot indicate where; you cannot say where he is. In that sense he is nowhere and in that sense he is everywhere. For the mind which lives in a space, it's very difficult to understand something beyond space. But whosoever follows the methods of Buddha and becomes a Master, immediately has a contact. Buddha still goes on guiding people who follow his path; Jesus still goes on guiding people who follow his path.

In Tibet there is a place on Kailash where, every year on the day Buddha left the world, the full moon night of Vaishakh, five hundred Masters gather together. Because this place, when five hundred Masters gather together every year, they have a realization of Buddha descending — again becoming visible.

This is an old promise, and Buddha still fulfills it. Five hundred Masters have to be there — not even a single less, because then it will not be possible. These five hundred Masters help as a weight, as an anchor, for Buddha to come down. Even a single Master less, and the phenomenon doesn't happen: because sometimes it was so — there were not five hundred Masters. Then that year there was no contact — no visible contact. Invisible contact remains, but no visible contact.

But Tibet has many Masters, and it was not a difficulty. Tibet is the most enlightened country; it has remained so up to now. It will not be so in the future, thanks to Mao. He has destroyed the whole subtle pattern that Tibet has created. The whole country was a monastery. In other countries monasteries exist; Tibet existed in the monastery.

And it was a rule that from every family one person has to take sannyas, become a lama, and this rule was made so that every year at least five hundred Masters are always available. When five hundred Masters gather together on Kailash just in the midnight — twelve o'clock — Buddha is again visible. He descends into time and space.

He has been guiding: every Master goes on guiding. Once you are near a Master, not near a teacher, you can trust. Even if you don't attain to enlightenment in this life, there will be a subtle guidance continuously for you — even if you don't realize that you are being guided.

Many Gurdjieff people have come to me. They have to come because Gurdjieff has been throwing them towards me. There is nobody else Gurdjieff can throw them or push them. And this is unfortunate, but this is so — that now there exists no Master in Gurdjieff's system, so he cannot make contact. Many Gurdjieff people will be coming sooner or later, and they are not aware because they cannot understand what is happening. They think this is just accidental.

If a Master exists on a certain path in time and space, then the original Master can go on sending instructions. And that's how religions have remained always alive. Once the chain is broken, the religion becomes dead. For example, Jaina religion has become dead because not a single Master is there with whom Mahavira can go on sending new instructions. Because with every age things change; mind changes, techniques have to be changed, methods have to be devised, new things have to be added, old things have to be deleted. Much work, every age needs.

If a Master exists on a certain path, then the original Master who is now a god can continue. But if the Master is not there on the earth, then the chain is broken and then the religion becomes dead. And it happens many times.

For example, Jesus never intended to create a new religion; he never thought about it. He was a Jew, and he was receiving direct instructions from old Jewish Masters who had become gods. But Jews won't listen to the new instructions. They will say, "This is not written in the scriptures. What are you talking about?" In the scriptures this is written, that if somebody hits you by a brick you throw a rock at him: eye for eye, life for life. And Jesus started saying that love your enemy — and if he hits on your one cheek give him the other.

It is not written in the Jewish scriptures, but this was the new instruction because the age has changed. This was a new method to work it out, and Jesus was receiving directly from gods — gods in Patanjali's sense: the old prophets. But that was not written in the scriptures. Jews killed him not knowing what they were doing. That's what Jesus said in the last moment, when he was on the cross he said, "God, forgive these people, because they don't know what they are doing. They are committing suicide. They are killing themselves, because they are breaking the link from their own Masters."

And that happened. The murder of Jesus became the greatest calamity for the Jews, and since two thousand years they have suffered because they have no contact. They live with the scriptures; they are the most scripture-oriented people on the earth. The Talmud, the Torah — they live with the scriptures and whenever an effort is made from the higher sources beyond time and space, they don't listen.

This has happened many times. That's how new religions are born. Unnecessary — there is no need! But the old people won't listen. They will say, "Where it is written?" It is not written. It is a new instruction, a new scripture. And if you don't listen to the new scripture, the new instruction will become a new religion. And see always the new religion seems to be more powerful than the old. Because it has latest instructions, can help man more.

Jews remained the same. Christianity spread to half the earth; now half of the world is Christian. Jainas have remained in India, a very small tiny minority because they won't listen. And they don't have any living Master. They have many *sadhus*, monks—many, because they can afford—they are a rich community— but not a single living Master. No instructions can be given through the higher sources. This was one of the greatest revelations of Theosophy in India—in this age, all over the world—that Masters continuously go on instructing. Patanjali says this is the third category of Masters: Master of Masters. This is what he means by a god.

> *Being beyond the limits of time, he is the Master of Masters.*

What is time and how one goes beyond time? Try to understand. Time is desire, because for desire time is needed. Time is a creation of desire. If you have no time, how can you desire? There is no space for desire to move. Desire needs future. That's why people who live with millions of desires are always afraid of death. Why are they afraid of death? Because death cuts time immediately. There is no time any more, and you have millions of desires, and here comes death.

Death means now no more future; death means now no more time. The clock may go on ticking, but you will not be ticking. And desire needs time to fulfill—future. You cannot be desirous in the present; there exists no desire in the present. Can you desire anything in the present? How you will desire it? Because immediately if you desire the future has entered. The tomorrow has come in or the next moment. How can you desire in this moment here now?

Desire is impossible without time — time is also impossible without desire — they are a phenomenon together, two aspects of the same coin. When one becomes desireless, one becomes timeless. Future stops, past stops. Only the present is there. When desire stops it is like as if a clock goes on ticking and the hands have been taken off. Just imagine a clock goes on ticking, and no hands, so you cannot say what is the time.

A man without desire is a clock ticking without hands. That is the state of a Buddha. In body, he lives, the clock goes on ticking, because the body has its own biological process to continue. It will be hungry, it will ask for food. It will be thirsty and ask for a drink. It will feel sleepy and will go to sleep. And the body will need, so it is ticking. But the innermost being has no time: the clock is without hands.

But because of the body you are anchored in the world — in that world of time. Your body has a weight, and because of that weight the gravitation still functions on you. When the body is left, when a Buddha leaves body, then the ticking itself stops. Then he is pure consciousness: no body, no hunger, no satiety; no body, no thirst; no body, then no need.

Remember this — desire and need — these two words. Desire is of the mind; need is of the body. Desire and need, then you are a clock with hands. Only need, no desire, then you are a clock without hands, and when need also drops, you have gone beyond time. This is eternity; beyond time is eternity.

For example: if I don't look at the watch — and I have to look continuously the whole day — if I don't look at the watch, I don't know what is the time. Even if I have seen it five minutes before, again I have to look because I don't know exactly, because now — no time inside — only the body is ticking.

Consciousness has no time. Time is created when

consciousness desires something: immediately time is created. In existence there is no time. If man is not there on the earth, time will disappear immediately. Trees tick, rocks tick. The sun will rise and the moon will set and everything will continue as it is, but there will be no time because time comes not with the present, it comes with the memory of past and the imagination of future.

A Buddha has no past. He is finished with it; he doesn't carry it. A Buddha has no future. He is finished with that also because he has no desire. But needs are there because the body is there. Few more karmas have to be fulfilled; few more days the body will go on ticking, just the old momentum will continue. You have to wind a clock. Even if you stop winding, it will continue to tick for few hours or few days. The old momentum will continue.

*Being beyond the limits of time, he is the Master of Masters.*

When need and desire both disappear, time disappears. And remember to make a distinction between desire and need; otherwise you can be in a very deep mess. Never try to drop needs. Nobody can drop, unless the body drops. And don't get confused what is what. Always remember what is need and what is desire.

Need comes from the body and desire comes from the mind. Need is animal; desire is human. Of course, when you feel hungry you need food. Stop when the need stops; your stomach immediately says, "Enough!" But the mind says, "A little more. It is so tasty." This is desire. Your body says, "I am thirsty," but the body never says for Coca Cola. The body says, "Thirsty"— you drink. You cannot drink water more than is needed, but Coca Cola you can drink more. It is a mind phenomenon.

Coca Cola is the only universal thing in this age — even in Soviet Russia. Nothing has entered, but Coca

Cola has entered. Even the iron curtain doesn't make any difference because human mind is human mind.

Always watch where need stops and desire starts. Make it a continuous awareness. If you can make the distinction, you have attained something — a clue to existence. Need is beautiful, desire is ugly. But there are people who go on desiring, and they go on cutting their needs. They are foolish, stupid! You cannot find more idiots in the world, because they are doing just the opposite.

There are people who will fast for days and desire for heaven. Fasting is cutting the need and desiring heaven is helping desire to be more there. They have a bigger time than yours, because they have to think of heaven — they have a vast time, heaven included in it. Your time stops at death. To you they will say, "You are a materialist." They are spiritualists because their time goes on and on. It covers heavens — not only one, seven — and even *moksha*, the final liberation, is within their time limit. They have a vast time, and you are materialists because your time stops at death.

Remember, it is easy to drop needs, because body is so silent you can torture it. And body is so adaptive that if you torture it too long it becomes adjusted to your torture. And it is dumb! It cannot say anything! If you fast, for two, three days it will say that "I am hungry, I am hungry!" But your mind is thinking of heaven, and without being hungry you cannot enter. It is written in the scriptures: "Fast" — so you don't listen to the body. It is also written in the scriptures that "Don't listen to the body; the body is the enemy."

And body is a dumb animal: you can go on torturing. For few days it will say, if you start a long fast, at the most the first week. . . Fifth, sixth day, the body stops because nobody is listening, so body starts making adjustments of its own. It has a reservoir for ninety days. Every healthy body has a reservoir of fat for ninety days for some emergency situation—not for fasting.

Sometime you are lost in a forest and you cannot get food. Sometime there is a famine and you cannot get food. For ninety days the body has a reservoir. It will feed itself; it eats itself. And it has a two-gear system. Ordinarily it asks for food. If you supply food, then the reservoir remains intact. If you don't supply, two, three days it goes on asking. If you still don't supply, it simply changes the gear. The gear is changed; then it starts eating itself.

That's why in fasting you lose one kilo weight every day. Where is this weight going? This weight is disappearing because you are eating your own fat, your own flesh. You have become a man-eater, a cannibal. Fasting is cannibalism. Within ninety days you will be a skeleton, every reservoir finished. Then you have to die.

It is easy to be violent to the body: it is so dumb. But to the mind it is difficult because mind is so vocal, it won't listen. And the real thing is to make the mind listen and cut the desires. Don't ask for heaven and paradise.

I was just reading a book on new religions in Japan. And as you know Japanese are so technically skilled people; they have created two paradises in Japan. Just to give you a glimpse, on a hill station they have made a small paradise—how it is up there... You just go and have a glimpse. A beautiful place they have made and absolutely clean they keep it—flowers and flowers and trees and shades and beautiful small bungalows, and they give you a glimpse of paradise so that you start desiring.

There is no paradise! Paradise is a creation of the mind. And there is no hell! That too is a creation of the mind. Hell is nothing but missing the paradise; that's all. And first you create, and then you miss because it is not there. And these people, these priests, the poisoners, they always help you to desire. First they create the desire; then follows the hell; then they come to save you.

Once I was passing through a very primitive road, and suddenly — and it was summer — I came on a path of road so muddy that I couldn't believe how this road has become so muddy. There has been no rain. But a patch almost of half a mile, but I thought it cannot be very deep so — I was driving the car — I went into it; then I was stuck. It was not only muddy, it has many holes. Then I waited if somebody comes to help, some truck.

A farmer came with a truck. When I asked him to help me, he said he will take twenty rupees. So I said, "Okay! You will take twenty rupees, but get me out of it." When I was out, I told the farmer that "At this price you must be doing the job day and night." He said, "No, not in the night, because I have to tote the water from the river for this road. Who do you think creates this mud here? And then I have to have a little sleep also because just early in the morning the business starts."

These are the priests. First they create mud: they tote water from the far-away river. And then you are bogged, and then they help you. There is no paradise and no hell, no heaven, no hell. You are being exploited, and you will be exploited unless you stop desiring.

A man who doesn't desire cannot be exploited. Then no priest can exploit, then no church can exploit him. It is because you desire, then you create the possibility of being exploited. Cut your desires as much as you can because they are unnatural. Never cut your needs because they are natural: fulfill your needs.

And look at the whole thing. Needs are not very many: they are not many at all. And they are so simple. What do you need? Food, water, a shelter, somebody to love you and somebody so that you can love him. What else you need? Love, food, shelter—simple needs. And all these needs, religions are against. Against love, they say practice celibacy. Against food, they say practice fasting. Against shelter, they say become monks, move, become wanderers—homeless. They are against needs. That's why they create a hell. And you are more and more in suffering, and more and more in their hands. Then you ask help, and the whole thing is a created thing.

Never go against needs, and always remember to cut desires. Desires are useless. What is a desire? It is not a desire of shelter. Desire is always for a better shelter. Desire is comparative, need is simple. You need a shelter, desire needs a palace. Need is very, very simple. You need a woman to love, a man to love. Desire? Desire needs a Cleopatra. Desire is simply for the impossible; need is for the possible. And if the possible is fulfilled, you are at ease. Even a Buddha needs that.

Desires are foolish. Cut desires and become aware. Then you will be beyond time. Desires create time; if you cut desires you will be beyond time. Bodily needs will remain til the body is there, but if desires disappear, then this is your last or, at the most last but one life. Soon you will also disappear. One who has attained desirelessness will sooner or later become beyond needs only because then the body is not needed. Body is a vehicle of the mind; if the mind is not there, body cannot be needed any more.

*He is known as Aum:*

And this God, the perfect flowering, is known as aum. Aum is the symbol of the universal sound. In you you hear thoughts, words, but never the sound of your being. When there is no desire, no need, when the body has dropped, when the mind disappears, what will happen? Then the real sound of the universe itself is heard. That is aum.

And all over the world people have realized this aum. Mohammedans, Christians, Jews, they call it amen. It is aum! Zoroastrians, Parsis, call it *ahura mazada*. That a and m — *ahura* is from a and *mazada* is from m — it is aum. They have made it a deity.

That sound is universal. When you stop, you hear it. Right now you are talking so much, chattering within yourself, you cannot hear it. It is a silent sound. It is so silent that unless you have completely stopped you will not be able to hear it. Hindus have called their gods a symbolic name — aum. Patanjali says, *He is known as Aum.* And if you want to find a Master, a Master of Masters, you will have to get more and more attuned to the sound of aum, oriented that he will not even leave a single word, and he will not use a single word more. . .

*Repeat and meditate. . .*

Wherever he says repeat aum, he always adds meditate. The difference has to be understood.

*Repeat and meditate on Aum.*

*Repeating and meditating on Aum brings about the disappearance of all obstacles and an awakening of a new consciousness.*

If you repeat and don't meditate, it will be Maharishi Mahesh Yogi's Transcendental Meditation — TM. If you repeat and don't meditate, then it is a hypnotic device. Then you fall into sleep. It is good because falling into sleep is beautiful. It is healthy: you will come out of it more calm. You will feel more well-being, more energy, more zest. But it is not meditation.

It is like a tranquilizer and a pep pill together. It gives you a good sleep, and then you feel in the morning very good. More energy is available, but it is not meditation, and it can become dangerous also if you use it for a long time. You can become addicted to it, and the more you use it, the more you will realize that there comes a point where you are stuck. Now, if you don't do it, you feel that you are missing something. If you do it, nothing happens.

This point has to be remembered: whenever meditating you feel that if you don't do it you miss it and if you do it nothing happens, then you are stuck. Then something is needed immediately to be done. It has become an addiction just like smoking cigarettes. If you don't smoke, you feel something is missing. You feel continuously that something has to be done; you feel restless. And if you smoke, nothing is gained. That is the definition of addiction. If something is gained, it is okay; but nothing is gained — it has become a habit. If you don't do, you feel miserable. If you do, no bliss comes out of it.

Repeat and meditate — repeat aum, aum, aum — and stand aloof from this repetition. Aum, aum, aum; the sound is all around you and you are alert, aware, watching, witnessing. That is meditating. Create the sound within you and still remain a watcher on the hill. In the valley, the sound is moving — aum, aum, aum — and you are standing above and watching, witnessing. If you don't watch, you will fall into sleep. It will be a hypnotic sleep. And Transcendental Meditation in the West is appealing people because they have lost the capacity to sleep well.

In India nobody bothers about Maharishi Mahesh Yogi because people are so fast asleep, snoring. They don't need it. But when a country becomes rich and people are not doing physical labor, the sleep is disturbed. Then either you take tranquilizer or TM. And TM is, of course, better because it is not so chemical. But it is still a very, very deep hypnotic device.

And hypnosis can be used in certain cases, but should not be made a habit, because ultimately it will give you a sleepy being. You will move as if in hypnosis; you will look like a zombie. You will not be aware and alert.

And the sound of aum is such a lullaby, because it is a universal sound. If you repeat it, you can completely become alcoholic through it, intoxicated. And then comes the danger, because the real thing is not to become intoxicated. The real thing is to become more and more aware. There are two possibilities you can drop out of your worries.

Psychoanalysts divide mind into three layers: first they call conscious, second they call the subconscious, third they call unconscious. Fourth they don't know yet —Patanjali calls superconscious. If you become more alert, you move above the conscious and reach the superconscious. That is the stage of a god—superconscious, super-aware.

But if you repeat a mantra without meditating, you fall into the subconscious. If you fall into the subconscious, it will give you good sleep, a well-being, health. But if you continue, you will fall into the unconscious, then you have become a zombie, and this is very, very bad—it is not good.

A mantra can be used as a hypnosis. If you are being operated in a hospital it is okay. Rather than taking chloroform, it is good to be hypnotized; it is less evil. If you don't feel sleepy, it is better to do TM than take a tranquilizer. It is less dangerous, less harmful. But it is not meditation.

So Patanjali continuously insists,

*Repeat and meditate on Aum.*

Repeat and create all around you the sound of aum, but don't be lost in it. It is such sweet sound, you will be lost. Remain alert—remain more and more alert! The more sound goes deeper, you become more and more alert; so the sound relaxes your nervous system, but not you. The sound relaxes your body, but not you. The sound sends your whole body and the physical system into sleep, but not you.

Then double process has started: the sound drops your body to a restful state and the awareness helps you to rise to the superconscious. Body moves to the unconscious, becomes a zombie, fast asleep, and you become a superconscious being. Then your body reaches to the bottom and you reach to the peak. Your body becomes the valley and you become the peak. And this is the point to be realized.

Repeat and meditate.

*Repeating and meditating on Aum brings about the disappearance of all obstacles and an awakening of new consciousness.*

The new consciousness is the fourth—the superconsciousness. But remember, only repetition is not good. Repetition is just to help to meditate. Repetition creates the object, the most subtle object is the sound of aum. And if you can be aware of the most subtle, your awareness also becomes subtle.

When you watch a gross thing, your awareness is gross. When you watch a sexual body, your awareness becomes sexual. When you watch something—an object for greed—your awareness becomes greed. Whatsoever you watch, you become. The observer becomes the observed: remember this.

Krishnamurti insists again and again the observer becomes the observed. Whatsoever you observe, you become. So if you observe the sound of aum, which is the deepest sound, the deepest music, the sound without sound, the sound which is uncreated—*anahat*, the sound which is just the nature of existence, if you become aware of it, you become that—you become a universal sound. The both, subject and object, meet and merge and become one. That is the superconscious where object and subject have dissolved, where the knower and the known are no more. Only one remains; the object and subject are bridged. This oneness is yoga.

The word yoga comes from the root *yuj*. It means meeting, combining together. It happens when subject and object are yoked together. The English word yoke also comes from *yuj*, the same root from where yoga comes. When subject and object are yoked together, sewed together so that they are no more separate, bridged, the gap disappears. You attain to a super-consciousness.

That's what Patanjali calls,

*Repeating and meditating on Aum brings about the disappearance of all obstacles and an awakening of a new consciousness.*

# The Beginning Of A New Path

The first question:

*Do you receive instructions from any Master of Masters?*

**I** AM NOT ON ANY ANCIENT path, so few things have to be understood. I am not like Mahavira who was the end of a long series of *Teerthankaras*, twenty-four—he was the twenty-fourth. In the past twenty-three had become Master of Masters, gods, on the same path, the same method, the same way of life, the same technique.

The first was Rishabh and the last was Mahavira. Rishabh had nobody in the past to look to. I am not like Mahavira, but like Rishabh. I am a beginning of a tradition, not the end. Many more will be coming on the same path. So I cannot look for instructions to anybody; that's not possible. A tradition is born and then a tradition dies, just as persons are born and persons die. I am the beginning, not the end. When somebody is in the middle of the series or at the end, he gets instructions from the Master of Masters.

The reason why I am not any path? I have worked with many Masters, but I have never been a disciple. I was a wanderer, wandering through many lives, criss-crossing many traditions, being with many groups, schools, methods, but never belonging to anybody. I was received with love, but I was never a part — a guest at the most, an overnight stay. That's why I learned so much. You cannot learn on one path so much; that's impossible.

If you move on one path, you know everything about it but nothing about anything else. Your whole being is absorbed in it. That has not been my way. I have been like a bee from one flower to another, gathering many fragrances. That's why I can be at ease with Zen, can be at ease with Jesus, can be at ease with Jews, can be at ease with Mohammedans, can be at ease with Patanjali — diverse ways, sometimes diametrically opposite.

But, to me, a hidden harmony exists. That's why people who follow one path are unable to understand me. They are simply baffled, bewildered. They know a particular logic, a particular pattern. If the thing fits into their pattern, it is right. If it doesn't fit, it is wrong. They have a very limited criterion. To me, no criterions exist. Because I have been with so many patterns, I can be at ease anywhere. Nobody is alien to me and I am not a stranger to anybody. But this creates a problem. I am not a stranger to anybody, but everybody becomes a stranger to me — has to be so.

If you belong not to a particular sect, then everybody thinks you as if you are the enemy. Hindus will be against me, Christians will be against me, Jews will be against me, Jains will be against me, and I am against nobody. Because they cannot find their pattern in me, they will be against me.

And I am talking about not pattern, but a deeper pattern which holds all the patterns. There is a pattern, another pattern, another pattern, millions of patterns. Then all the patterns are held by something under-ground which is the pattern of patterns — the hidden harmony. They cannot look at it, but they are not at fault also. When you live with a certain tradition, a certain philosophy, a certain way of looking at things, you become attuned to it.

In a way, I was never attuned to anybody — not that much so that I could have become a part of them. In a sense it is a misfortune, but in another sense it proved a blessing. Many who worked with me achieved liberation before me. It was a misfortune to me. I lagged and lagged behind because never working totally with anything, moving from one to another.

Many achieved who started with me. Even few who started after me achieved before me. This was a misfortune, but in another sense this has been a blessing because I know every home. I may not belong to any home, but I am at home everywhere. That is why I have got no Master of Masters — I was never a disciple. To be directed by a Master of Masters, you have to be a disciple to a certain Master. Then you can be directed. Then you know the language. So I am not directed by anybody but helped by many. The difference has to be understood: not directed, I don't receive any orders, "Do this or don't do that", but helped by many.

Jains may not feel that I belong to them, but Mahavira feels, because at least he can see the pattern of patterns. Followers of Jesus may not be able to understand me, but Jesus can. So I am helped by many. That's why many people are coming to me from different sources. You cannot find such a gathering anywhere on the earth at this time. Jews are there, Christians are there, Mohammedans are there, Hindus, Jains, Buddhists, from all over the world. And more, many more, will be coming soon.

That's a help from many Masters. They know I can be helpful to their disciples; they will be sending many more — but no instructions, because I never received instructions from any Master as a disciple. Now there is no need also. Just a help, and that is better; I feel more at freedom. Nobody can be so free as I am.

Because if you receive directions from Mahavira, you cannot be as free as I am. A Jain has to remain Jain. He has to go on talking against Buddhism, against Hinduism. He has to because it is a fight of many patterns and traditions. And traditions have to fight if they want to survive. And for the sake of disciples they have to be argumentative; they have to say, "That is wrong," because only then the disciple can feel that "This is right." Against wrong, the disciple feels what is right.

With me you will be at a loss. If you are just here with your intellect, you will be confused. You will go crazy because this moment I say something and next moment I contradict it: because this moment I was talking about one tradition, another moment I am talking about another. And sometimes I am not talking about any tradition; I am talking about me. Then you cannot find it anywhere in any scripture.

But I am helped, and the help is beautiful because I am not supposed to follow it. I am not forced to follow it. It is up to me. Help is given unconditionally. If I feel like doing it, I will do; if I don't feel, I will not do it. I have no obligation to anybody.

But if you become some day enlightened, then you can receive. If I am not in the body, then you can receive instructions from me. This always happens to the first person, when a tradition starts. It is a beginning, a birth, and you are near a birth process. And it is most beautiful when something is born, because it is most alive. By and by, as a child grows, the child is coming nearer and nearer to death. A tradition is freshest when it is born. It has a beauty of its own—incomparable, unique.

The people who listened to Rishabh, the first Jain *Teerthankara*, had a different quality. When they listened to Mahavira, it was thousands of years old. It was just on the verge of dying. With Mahavira, it died.

When in a tradition no more Masters are born, it is dead. It means the tradition is no more growing. Jains closed. With the twenty-fourth they said, "Now, no more Masters, no more *Teerthankaras.*" To be with Nanak was beautiful because something new was coming out of the womb — the womb of the universe. Just as you watch a child being born — a mystery — an unknown penetrating the known, the bodiless becoming the embodied. It is fresh like dewdrops. Soon everything will be covered with dust. Soon, as time passes, things will become old.

But by the time of the tenth guru of the Sikhs, the tenth Master, things became dead. Then they closed the line and they said, "Now no more Masters. Now the scripture itself will be the Master." That's why they called their scripture "Guru-granth" — the Master scripture. Now no more persons will be there; just a dead scripture will be the Master now. And when a scripture is dead, it is futile — not only futile: it is poisonous. Don't allow anything dead in your body. It will create poison; it will destroy your whole system.

Here, something new is born, a beginning. It is fresh, but that's why it is very difficult also to see it. Because if you go to the Ganges, the source of the Ganges, it is so tiny there — fresh, of course: never again it will be so fresh, because when it moves it gathers many things, accumulates, becomes more and more dirty. At Kashi it is the dirtiest, but then you call it "Holy Ganges" because now it is so vast. It has accumulated so much, now even a blind man can see it. At the Gangotri — at the beginning, at the source — you need to be very perceptive. Only then you can see; otherwise it is just a trickling of drops. You cannot even believe that this trickling of the drops is going to become Ganges — unbelievable.

It is difficult right now to see what is happening because it is a very, very tiny stream, just like a child. People missed with Rishabh, the first Jain *Teerthankara*, but they could recognize Mahavira — see? Jains don't think much of the first — Rishabh. In fact, they pay their whole homage to Mahavira. In fact, in the western mind, Mahavira is the originator of Jainism. Because they pay so much respect to Mahavira in India, that how others can feel that somebody else was the originator? Rishabh has become legendary, forgotten; may have been, may not have been, he doesn't seem to be historical — hoary past — and you don't know much about him. Mahavira is historical, and he is the Ganges, near Benares, Kashi — so vast.

Remember that the beginning is small, but never again the mystery will be so deep as in the beginning. The beginning is life and the end is death. With Mahavira, death enters into Jain tradition. With Rishabh, life entered, came down from the above Himalayas, to the earth.

I have got nobody to be responsible to, nobody to get instructions from, but much help is available. And if you take it in its totality, then it is more than any single Master can instruct. When I am talking about Patanjali, Patanjali is helpful. I can talk exactly as if he was talking here. I am not talking, in fact; these are not commentaries. It is he himself using me as a vehicle. When I am talking about Heraclitus, he is there — but as a help. This you have to understand, and become more perceptive so that you can see the beginning.

To move into a tradition when it has become a great force does not take much perceptivity, much sensitivity. To come when things are beginning, just in the morning, is difficult. By the evening many come, but then they come because the thing has become so vast and powerful. In the morning only those few chosen come who have the sensitivity to feel that something great is being born. You cannot prove it right now. Time will prove it. It will take thousands of years to prove what was being born, but you are fortunate to be here. And don't miss the opportunity, because this is the freshest point and the most mysterious.

If you can feel it, if you can allow it to go deep into you, many things will become possible in a very short period of time. It is yet not respectable to be with me; it is not a prestige. In fact, only gamblers can be with me who do not bother and worry about what others say. People who are respectable cannot come. After a few years, when the tradition becomes by and by dead, it becomes respectable. Then people will come, but those will be dead people. They will come only when something becomes respectable. They will come because of the ego.

You are here not because of the ego, because with me there is nothing to gain for the ego at least. You will lose. With Rishabh, only people who were alive and courageous and daring, adventurous, they moved; with Mahavira, dead businessmen — not gamblers. That is why Jains have become a business community. The whole community is business community; they don't do anything except business. Business is the least courageous thing in the world. That's why businessmen become cowards. In the first place they were cowards; that's why they became businessmen.

A farmer is more courageous because he lives with the unknown, does not know what is going to happen, whether rains will be there or not — nobody knows. And how can you believe on the clouds? You can believe on the banks, but you cannot believe on the clouds. Nobody knows what is going to happen; he hangs with the unknown. But he lives a more courageous life — a warrior.

Mahavira himself was a warrior; all the twenty-four *Teerthankaras* of the Jains were warriors. Then what misfortune happened? What happened that the whole followers became businessmen? They became businessmen with Mahavira because they came only with Mahavira — when the tradition was glorious, had a legendary past, become already a myth and was respectable to be with.

Dead people come only when something becomes dead; alive people come only when something is alive. Younger people will be coming to me more. Even if somebody old comes to me, he is bound to be younger in the heart. Old people look for prestige, respect. They will go to dead churches and temples where nothing is except emptiness and a past. What is past?—an emptiness. Anything alive is herenow, and anything alive has a future, because future grows out of it. The moment you start looking at the past, there can be no growth.

*Do you receive instructions from any Master of Masters?* No! But I receive help which is more beautiful. And I have been a loner, a vagabond with no home, passing, learning, moving, never staying anywhere. So I have nobody to look up to. If I had to find something, I had to find it myself. Much help available, but I had to work it out. And in a way that is going to be a great help because then I don't depend on any code. I watch the disciple. There is nobody as a Master to me to look to. I have to look at the disciple more deeply to find the clue. What will help you, I have to look into you. That's why my teaching, my methods, differ with each disciple. I have no universal formula, cannot have; no fixed rules, I have to respond. I have not a discipline already— ready-made. Rather, a growing phenomenon. Every disciple adds to it. When I start working with a new disciple, I have to look into him, seek, find what will help him, how he can grow. And each time, with each disciple, a new code is born.

You are going really in a mess when I am gone— because there will be so many stories from each disciple, and you will not be able to make any end, head or tail of it—because I am talking to each individual as individual. The system is growing through him, and it is growing in many, many directions. It is a vast tree, many branches, many sub-branches, going in all directions.

I don't receive any instructions from the Masters. I receive instructions from you. When I look into you, in your unconscious, in your depth, I receive instructions from there and I work it out for you. It is always a new response.

The second question:

*Why do Masters need directions from Master of Masters? Are they not enough in themselves when they have reached enlightenment? Or are there stages of enlightenment too?*

No, there are not stages in fact, but when a Master is in the body, and when the Master leaves the body and becomes bodiless, there is a difference—not exactly stages. It is just like you are standing by the side of the road under a tree: you can see a patch of the road; beyond that patch you cannot see. Then you climb up the tree. You remain the same; nothing is happening to you or your consciousness. But you climb up the tree, and from the tree now you can look miles to this side and miles to that.

Then you fly in an airplane. Nothing has happened to you; your consciousness remains the same. But now you can see for thousands of miles. In the body you are on the road—by the side of the road—encased in the body. The body is the lowest point in existence because it means committed to the matter still, being with the matter still. Matter is the lowest point and God is the highest point.

When a Master attains to enlightenment in the body, the body has to fulfill its karmas, the past *samskaras*, the past conditionings. Every account has to be closed; only then can the body be left. It is like this: your airplane has arrived, but you have many businesses to finish. All the creditors are there, and they are asking to close the account before you leave. And there are many credits, because many lives you have been promising,

doing things, acting, behaving, sometimes good, sometimes bad, sometimes a sinner, sometimes a saint. You
have accumulated much! Before you leave, the whole
existence demands you to complete everything.

When you have become enlightened, now you know
that you are not the body, but you owe many things to
the body and the material world. Time is needed—
Buddha lived forty years after his enlightenment, Mahavira also lived near about forty years—to pay, to pay
everything that they owe, to complete every circle that
they started. No new action, but the old hanging things
have to be finished, the old hangover has to be finished.
When all the accounts are closed, now you can take
your aircraft.

Up to now, with matter, you have been moving hori-
zontally—just like in a bullock cart. Now you can move
vertically. Now you can go upwards. Before this, you
have always been going forwards or backwards; there
was no vertical movement. And the higher you rise—
and the God is the highest point, the Master of Masters
—from where the perception is total. Your consciousness is the same; nothing has changed: an enlightened
man has the same consciousness as the supreme state of
consciousness, God—no difference of consciousness.
But the perception, the field of perception, is different;
now he can look everywhere.

There was a great debate in the times of Buddha and
Mahavira. It will be useful to understand it at this point
for this question. There was a debate: followers of
Mahavira used to say that Mahavira is omnipotent,
omniscient, omnipresent, *sarvagya*, all-knowing. In a
way they are right, because once you are freed from
matter and body you *are* God. But in a way they were
wrong, because you may be freed from the body, but
you have yet not left it. The identification is broken;
you know that you are not the body. But still you are
in it.

It is as if you live in a house; then suddenly you come

to know that this house doesn't belong to you—somebody else's house and you were living in it. But then too, to leave the house you will have to make arrangements, you will have to remove things. And it will take time. You know this house is not yours; your attitude has changed. Now you are not worried about this house, what happens to it. If next day it falls and becomes a ruins, it is nothing to you. If next day you leave and it takes fire, it is nothing to you: it belongs to somebody else. Just a moment before, you were identified with the house; it was your house. If there was fire, if the house fell down, you would have much worried. Now the identification is broken.

Mahavira's followers are right in a sense, because when you have come to know yourself, you have become all-knowing. But Buddha's followers used to say that this is not right—a Buddha can know if he wants to know something, but he is not all-knowing. They used to say that if the Buddha wants, he can focus his attention in any direction, and wherever he focuses his attention, he will be able to know. He is capable of omniscience, but not omniscient. The difference is subtle, delicate, but beautiful. Because they said if he knows everything and all things continuously, he will go mad. This body cannot bear that much.

They are also right. A Buddha in the body can know anything if he wants to know. His consciousness, because of the body, is like a torch. You go in the dark with the torch. You can know anything if you focus; light is with you. But a torch is a torch; it is not a flame. A flame will give light in all directions; a torch focuses in a particular direction—wherever you want. The torch has no choice! You can look to the north, and then it will reveal the north. You can look to the south, and then it will reveal the south. But all the four directions are not revealed together. If you move the torch to the south, then the north is closed. It is a narrow flow of light.

This was Buddha's followers' standpoint. And Mahavira's followers used to say that he is not like a torch, he is like a lamp; all directions are revealed. But I favor Buddha's followers' standpoint. When the body is there, you are narrowed down. Body is a narrowing. You become like a torch—because you cannot see from the hands, you can see only from the eyes. If you can see only from the eyes, you cannot see from your back because you don't have any eyes there. You have to move your head.

With the body everything is focused and narrow. The consciousness is unfocused and flowing in all directions, but the vehicle, the body, is not in all directions—it always focused, so your consciousness also becomes narrowed down to it. But when the body is no more there, and a Buddha has left the body, then there is no problem. All directions are revealed together.

That's the point to be understood. That's why even an enlightened person can be guided, because an enlightened person is still tethered to the body, anchored in the body, in the narrow body, and a god is unanchored, floating in the highest sky. From there he can see all directions. From there he can see the past, the future, the present. From there his view is unclouded. That's why he can help.

Your view, even if you become enlightened in the body, is clouded. The body is there all around you. The status of consciousness is the same, the innermost reality of the consciousness is the same, the quality of the light is the same. But one light is tethered to the body and has become narrow; one light is not tethered to anything at all—just a floating light. In the highest of skies, guidance is possible.

*Why do Masters need directions from a Master of Masters?*

That's the reason.

*Are they not enough in themselves when they
have reached enlightenment or are there stages
of enlightenment too?*

They are enough! They are enough to guide disciples;
they are enough to help disciples. Nothing is needed.
But still they are tethered, and one who is untethered is
always a good help. You cannot look in all directions;
he can look.

You can also move and look, but that has to be done.
This is what I am doing: having no instructor above,
nobody to guide me, I have to be continuously on move
—looking from this direction and that, watching from
this direction and that, looking at you through many
standpoints so that your totality can be looked. I can
look through, but I have to be moving around you. Just
a glance will not help because a glance will be narrowed
through the body. I am having a torch and moving all
around you, looking from every standpoint possible.

In a way it is difficult because I have to work more.
In a way it is very beautiful because I have to work
more and I have to look from every standpoint possible. I come to know many things which ready-made
instructions cannot do. And when the Master of Masters in Patanjali's ideology—a god—gives instructions,
he gives no explanations; he gives simply instructions.
He simply says, "Do this; don't do that."

Those who follow these instructions, they will also
look like ready-made. It is bound to be so because they
will say, "Do this." They will not have the explanation.
And very coded instructions are given. Explanations are
very difficult—and there is no need also for them, because when it is given from a higher standpoint it is
okay. Just one has to be obedient.

The Master is obedient to the Master of Masters, and
you have to be obedient to the Master. An obedience
follows. It is just like a military hierarchy: not much
freedom. Much is not allowed! Order is order! If you

ask for explanation, you are rebellious. And this is the problem, one of the greatest problems humanity has to face now: now man cannot be obedient as in the past. You cannot simply say, "Don't do this"; explanation is needed. And not any ordinary explanation will do. A very authentic explanation is needed because the very mind of humanity is no more obedient. Now rebelliousness is built in; a child is born rebellious now.

It was totally different in the days of Buddha and Mahavira. Everybody is taught to be individual, to stand on his own, to believe in himself. Trust has become difficult. Obedience is not possible. If somebody follows without asking, you think he is a blind follower. He is condemned. Now only a Master can help you who has all the explanations—more than you require, who can exhaust you completely. You go on asking; he can go on answering you. A moment comes when you are tired of asking, and you say, "Okay, I will follow."

Never before this it was so. It was simple: when Mahavira says, "Do this," you do this. But this is not possible, simply because man is so different. The modern mind is a rebellious mind, and you cannot change it. This is how evolution has brought it to be, and nothing is wrong in it. That is why old Masters are falling off the road; nobody listens to them. You go to them. They have instructions, beautiful instructions, but they don't provide any explanation, and now the first thing is explanation. The instruction should follow as a syllogism. All explanations should be given first, and then the Master should say, "Therefore, do this."

It is a lengthy process, but it's how it is. Nothing can be done. And in a sense it is a beautiful growth, because when you simply trust, your trust has no salt in it, no tension in it. Your trust has no sharpness in it. It is a hodge-podge thing—shapeless: no tonality in it, no color in it. It is just grey. But when you can doubt, you can argue, you can reason and a Master can satisfy all your reasons and arguments and doubts, then arises a trust which has a beauty of its own because against the background of doubt it has been achieved.

Against all doubts it has been achieved, against all challenges it has been achieved. It has been a fight. It was not simple and cheap: it has been costly. And when you achieve something after a long fight, it has a meaning of its own. If you simply get it on the road it just lying there and take it home, it has no beauty. If Kohinoors are there all over the earth, who will bother to take them home? If a Kohinoor is just an ordinary pebble lying anywhere, then who will bother?

In the old days, faith was like pebbles all over the earth. Now it has to be a Kohinoor. Now it has to be a precious achievement. Instructions won't help. A Master has to be so deep in his explanations that he exhausts you. I never say to you don't ask. In fact, just otherwise is the case. I say to you ask, and you don't find questions.

I will bring all the questions possible from your unconscious to the surface, and I will solve them. Nobody can say to you that you are a blind follower. And I will not give you a single instruction without totally satisfying your reason — no, because that is not going to help you in any way.

Instructions are given from the Masters of Masters, but they are just quoted words — sutras: "Do this; don't do that." In the new age, that won't help. Man is so rational now that even if you are teaching irrationality you have to reason it about. That's what I am doing: teaching you the absurdity, the irrational, teaching you the mysterious — and through reason. Your reason has to be so much used that you yourself become aware that this is futile — throw it. You have to be so much talked about your reason that you get fed up with it: you drop it on your own, not through instruction.

Because instruction can be given, but you will cling.

That won't help. I'm not going to say to you, "Just trust me." I'm creating the whole situation in which you cannot do otherwise. You will have to trust. It will take a time—a little longer—than simple obedience. But it is worth.

The third question:

*We, in our unawareness and egoistic state, are not always in touch with the Master. But is the Master always in touch with us?*

Yes, because a Master is in touch with all the four layers of you. Your conscious layer is only one of the four layers. But that is possible only when you have surrendered and accepted him as your Master—not before that. If you are just a student, learning, then when you are in touch, the Master is in touch; when you are not in touch, he is also not in touch.

Has to be understood, this phenomenon. . . You have four minds: the supermind which is the possibility of the future, of which only seeds you carry—nothing has sprouted—only seeds, just the potentiality. Then the conscious mind—a very small fragment with which you reason, think, decide, argue, doubt, believe—this conscious mind is in touch with a Master to whom you have not surrendered. So whenever this is in touch, the Master is in touch. If this is not in touch, then the Master is not in touch. You are a student, and you have not taken the Master as a Master. You still think about him as a teacher.

Teacher and student exist in the conscious mind. Nothing can be done because you are not open; your all three doors are closed. Superconscious is just a seed; you cannot open its doors.

Subconscious is just below the conscious. That is possible if you love. If you are here with me only because of your reasoning, your conscious door is open. Whenever you open it, I am there. If you don't open it, I am outside; I cannot enter. Just below the conscious is the subconscious. If you are in love with me — not just a teacher and a student relationship but more intimate, a love-like phenomenon — then the subconscious door is open. Many times the conscious door will be closed by you. You will argue against me; you will be sometimes negative; sometimes you will be against me. But that doesn't matter. The unconscious door of love is open, and I can always remain in touch with you.

But that too is not a perfect door because sometimes you can hate me. If you hate me, you have closed that door also. Love is there, but the opposite, hate, is also there; it is always with love. The second door will be more open than the first — because the first changes its moods as fast that you don't know. . . Any moment it goes on changing. Just one moment it was here, the next moment it is not there; it is a momentary phenomenon.

Love is a little longer. It also changes its moods, but its moods have longer periods. Sometimes you will hate me. In thirty days almost there will be eight days — one week and four days, you will hate me. But three weeks it is open. With the reason, a week is too long; it is an eternity. With the reason, one moment here, another moment against: for, against, it goes on. If the second door is open and you are in love with me, even if the door with reason is closed, I can remain in contact.

The third door is below subconscious: that is the unconscious. Reason opens the first door — if you feel convinced with me. Love opens the second door which is bigger than the first — if you are in love with me: not convinced, but in love — feeling an affinity, a harmony, an affection.

The third door opens by surrender, if you are initiated by me, if you have taken the jump into sannyas, if you have taken a jump and said to me, "Now — now you be my mind. Now you take the reins of me. Now you guide me and I will follow." Not that you will always be able to do it, but just the very gesture that you surrendered opens the third door.

The third door remains open. You may be against me rationally. It doesn't matter: I am in touch. You may hate me. It doesn't matter: I am in touch — because the third door always remains open. You have surrendered. And it is very difficult to close the third door — very, very difficult! It is difficult to open, it is difficult to close. It is difficult to open, but not as difficult as to close it. But that too can be closed because you have opened it. That too can be closed! You can decide someday to take your surrender back. Or, you can go and surrender yourself to somebody else. But that never — almost never — happens, because with these three doors the Master is working to open the fourth door.

So there is very. . .almost impossible possibility that you will take your surrender back. Before you have taken it, he must have opened the fourth door which is beyond you. You cannot open it, you cannot close it. The door that you open, you remain the master to close it also. But the fourth has nothing to do with you. That is the superconscious. All these three doors are needed to open so the Master can forge a key for the fourth door, because you don't have the key, otherwise you yourself can open it. The Master has to forge; it is a forgery because the owner himself doesn't have the key.

The whole effort of a Master is to have enough time from these three doors to enter to the fourth and forge a key and open it. Once it is opened, you are no more. You cannot do anything now. You may close all the three doors — he has the key for the fourth and he is always in contact. Then even if you die, it doesn't matter. You go to the very end of the earth, you go the moon, does not make any difference; he has the key for the fourth. And, in fact, a real Master never keeps the key. He simply opens the four and throws the key in the ocean. So there is no possibility to steal it or do anything—nothing!

I have forged a fourth-door key of many of you and have thrown it, so don't unnecessarily trouble yourself; it is futile, now nothing can be done. Once the fourth is opened, then there is no problem. All the problems exist before it, because at the very last moment the Master was getting ready the key because the key is difficult. . .

For millions of lives the door has remained closed; it has gathered all sorts of rust. It looks like a wall, not like a door. It is difficult to find where the lock is—and everybody has a separate lock, so there is no master key. One key won't help because everybody is as individual as your thumbprint. Nobody has that print anywhere—not in the past, never in the future. Your thumbprint will be simply yours, a single phenomenon. It never is repeated.

Your inner lock is also like your thumbprint—absolutely individual: no master key can help. That's why a Master is needed, because master key cannot be purchased. Otherwise, once a key is made, everybody's door can be opened. No, everybody has a separate type of door, a separate type of lock—his own locking system—and you have to watch and find and forge a key, a special key for it.

Once your fourth door is open, then the Master is in constant touch with you. You may forget him completely: it makes no difference. You may not remember him: it makes no difference. The Master leaves the body: it makes no difference. Wherever he is, wherever you are, the door is open. And this door exists beyond time and space. That's why it is the supermind: it is superconscious.

*We in our unawareness and our egoistic state are not always in touch with the Master, but is the Master always in touch with us?*

Yes, but only when the fourth door is opened. Otherwise, with the third door, he is more or less in contact. With the second door, half time almost in contact. With the first door, only momentarily in contact.

So allow me to open your fourth door—and the fourth door is opened in a certain moment. That moment is when all your three doors are open. Even if a single door is closed, the fourth cannot be opened. It is a mathematical puzzle. And this condition is needed: your first, conscious door is open; your second door is open—your subconscious, your love—you have surrendered, you have taken a step into initiation, your third, unconscious door is open.

When all the three doors are open, when in a certain moment all the three doors are open, the fourth can be opened. So it happens that while you are awake, the fourth is difficult to open. While you are asleep, only then. So my real work is not in the day. It is in the night when you are fast asleep snoring, because then you don't create any trouble. You are so fast asleep, you don't reason against. You have forgotten about reasoning.

In deep sleep, your heart functions well. You are more loving than when you are awake, because when you are awake many fears surround you. And because of fear love is not possible. When you are fast asleep, fears disappear, love flowers. Love is a nightflower. You must have watched night queen—the flower that flowers in the night. Love is a night queen. It flowers in the night—because of you; there is no other reason. It can flower in the day, but then you have to change yourself. Tremendous change is needed before the love can flower in the day.

That's why you see that when people are intoxicated they are more loving. Go into any tavern where people have drunk too much: they are almost always loving. See two drunkards moving on the street hanging on each other's shoulder: so loving—as if one! They are asleep.

When you are not afraid, love flowers. Fear is the poison. And when deep down in sleep, you are already surrendered because sleep is a surrender. And if you have surrendered to a Master, he can enter into your sleep. You will not be even able to hear his footsteps. He can enter silently and work. It is a forgery, just like thieves enter in the night when you are asleep. A Master is a thief. When you are fast asleep and you don't know what is happening, he enters in you and opens the fourth.

Once the fourth is opened, then there is no problem. Every effort and every trouble that you can create, you can create only before the fourth is open. The fourth is a point of no return. Once the fourth is open, the Master can twenty-four hours be with you — there is no problem.

The last question:

*How can one cut desires without suppressing them?*

Desires are dreams: they are not realities. You cannot fulfill them and you cannot suppress them, because to fulfill a certain thing it needs to be real; to suppress a certain thing also needs to be real. Needs can be fulfilled and needs can be suppressed. Desires neither can be fulfilled nor can be suppressed. Try to understand this because this is very complex.

A desire is a dream. If you understand this, it disappears. No need to suppress it. What is the need to suppress a desire? You want to become very famous: this is a dream, a desire, because the body doesn't bother to be famous. In fact the body suffers very much when you become famous. You don't know how the body suffers when a person becomes famous. Then there is no peace. Then continuously you are bothered, troubled by others because you are so famous.

Somewhere Voltaire has written that "When I was not famous, I used to pray to God every night that 'Make me famous. I am nobody, so make me somebody.' And then I become famous. Then I started to pray, 'Enough is enough: now make me again a nobody' — because before I used to go on the streets of Paris and nobody will look at me and I felt so sad. Nobody would pay any attention to me — as if I didn't exist at all. I will move into the restaurants, come out; nobody, even the waiters will not pay attention to me."

What about kings? They didn't know that Voltaire existed. "Then I became famous," he writes. "Then it was difficult to move from the streets because people will gather. It was difficult to go anywhere. It was difficult to go in a restaurant and take food at rest. A crowd will gather."

A moment came when it was almost impossible for him to get out of the house because in those days there was a superstition in Paris, in France, that if you can get a piece of cloth from a very famous man and can make a locket out of it, it is a luck. So wherever he will go, he will come naked because people will tear his clothes — and they will harm his body also. When he used to come from some other town back to Paris, or will go, police was needed to bring him home.

So he used to pray that "I was wrong. You simply make me again a nobody, because I cannot go and watch the river. I cannot go out and see the sunrise, I cannot go to the hills, I cannot move. I have become a prisoner."

Those who are famous are always prisoners. Body doesn't need to be famous; body is so absolutely okay, it needs nothing like such nonsense things. It needs simple things — food; it needs water to drink; it needs a shelter when it is too hot, to come under: its needs are very, very simple. The world is mad because of desires, not because of needs. And people go mad! They go on cutting down their needs, and growing and increasing their desires. There are people who would like to drop one meal per day, but they cannot drop their newspaper, they cannot drop going to the cinema, they cannot drop smoking. They can drop food — needs can be dropped — desires cannot be. The mind has become a despot.

Body is always beautiful: remember it. This is one of the basic rules I give to you — a rule unconditionally true, absolutely true, categorically true: body is always beautiful, mind is ugly. It is not the body that has to be changed. There is nothing to change in it. It is the mind! And mind means desiring. The body needs, but body needs are real needs.

If you want to live, you need food. Fame is not needed to live, respect is not needed to be alive. You need not be a very great man or a very great painter — famous, known to the whole world. You need not be a Nobel Prize winner to live, because Nobel Prize doesn't fulfill any need in the body.

If you want to drop needs, you will have to suppress them — because they are real! If you fast, you have to suppress hunger. Then there is suppression, and every suppression is wrong because suppression is a fight inside, and you are wanting to kill the body, and the body is your anchor, your ship which will lead you to the other shore. Body keeps the treasure, the seeds of divine within you, protected. Food is needed for that protection, water is needed, shelter is needed, comfort is needed — for the body, because the mind doesn't want any comfort.

Look at the modern furniture: it is not comfortable at all, but the mind says, "This is modern, and what are you doing sitting in an old chair? The world has changed and the modern furniture has come." The modern furniture is really weird. You feel uncomfortable in it; you cannot sit in it long. But it is modern! The mind says modern must be there because how can you be out of date? Be up to date!

Modern dresses are uncomfortable, but they are modern, and the mind says that you have to be with the fashion. And man has done so many ugly things because of fashion. Body needs nothing: these are mind needs, and you cannot fulfill them — never, because they are unreal! Only unreality cannot be fulfilled. How can you fulfill an unreal need which is not there in fact? What is the need of fame? Just meditate on it. Close your eyes and look. Where it is needed in the body? How it will help if you are famous? Will you be more healthy if you are famous? Will you be more silent, peaceful, if you are famous? What you will gain out of it?

Always make the body the criterion. Whenever the mind says something, ask the body, "What do you say?" And if the body says foolish, drop it. And there is no suppression in it because it is an unreal thing. How can you suppress an unreal thing? In the morning, you get out of bed and you remember a dream. Have you to suppress it or you have to fulfill it? Because in the dream, you dreamed that you have become the emperor of the whole earth. Now what to do? Should you try? Otherwise the question arises, "If we don't try, then it is a suppression." But a dream is a dream! How can you suppress a dream? A dream disappears by itself. You have to be only aware. You have to only know that it is a dream. When a dream is a dream and known as such, it disappears.

Try to find out what is a desire and what is a need. Need is body oriented; desire has no orientation in the body. It has no roots. It is just a floating thought in the mind. And almost always your body needs come from your body and your mind needs come from others. Somebody purchases a beautiful car. Somebody else has purchased a beautiful car, an imported car, and now your mind need arises. How can you tolerate this?

Mulla Nasruddin was driving the car and I was sitting with him. The moment we entered the neighborhood — it was a very hot summer day — he immediately closed all the windows of the car. I said, "What are you doing?" He said, "What do you mean? Should I let my neighborhood people know that I don't have an air-conditioned car?"

Perspiring, I also perspired with him. It was like an oven, hot, but how can you allow your neighbors to know that you don't have an air-conditioned car? This is a mind need. The body says, "Drop it! Are you mad?" It is perspiring. It is saying, "No!" Listen to the body; don't listen to the mind. Mind's needs are created by others all around you; they are foolish, stupid, idiotic.

Body needs are beautiful, simple. Fulfill body needs; don't suppress them. If you suppress them, you will become more and more ill and diseased. Never bother about the mind needs; once you know that this is a mind need. . .and is there much difficulty to know? What is the difficulty? It is so simple to know that this is a mind need. Simply ask the body; inquire in the body; go find the root. Is there any root for it?

You will look foolish. Your all kings and emperors are foolish. They are clowns: just see. Dressed with thousands of medals, they look foolish! What they are doing? And for this they have suffered long. To attain this, they have passed through so many miseries and still they are miserable. They have to be miserable. Mind is the door to hell, and the door is nothing but desire. Kill desires. You will not find any blood coming out of them because they are bloodless.

But kill a need, and there will be bloodshed. Kill a need, and you will die in part. Kill a desire; you will not die. Rather, on the contrary, you will become freer. More freedom will come out of dropping desires. If you can become a man of need and no desires, you are already on the path and the heaven is not far off.

# The
# Obstacles
# To
# Meditation

*Disease, languor, doubt, carelessness, laziness,
sensuality, delusion, impotency and instability are the
obstacles that distract the mind.*

*Anguish, despair, tremors and irregular breathing are
the symptoms of a distracted mind.*

*To remove these, meditate on one principle.*

**P**ATANJALI BELIEVES – AND
not only believes, he knows also
– that sound is the basic element
of existence. Just as physicists
say that electricity is the basic
element, yogis say that sound is the basic
element. They agree with each other in a
subtle way.

Physicists say that sound is nothing but a modification of electricity and yogis say that electricity is
nothing but a modification of sound. Then both are
true. Sound and electricity are two forms of one phenomenon, and to me, that phenomenon is not known
yet and will not be known ever. Whatsoever we know
will be just a modification of it. You may call it electricity, you may call it sound, you may call it fire like
Heraclitus, you may call it water like Lao Tzu: that

depends on you. But all these are modifications — forms of the formless. That formless will always remain unknown.

How can you know the formless? Knowledge is possible only when there is a form. When something becomes visible, then you can know it. How can you make invisibility the object of knowledge? The very nature of invisibility is that it cannot be objectified. You cannot pinpoint it — where it is, what it is. Only something visible can become the object.

So whenever anything is known, it will be just a modification of the unknown. The unknown remains unknown. It is unknowable. So it depends on you what you call it, and it depends on the utility you are going to put it to. For the yogi, electricity is not relevant. He is working in the inner lab of being. There, sound is more relevant, because through sound he can change many phenomena inside and through sound he can change the inner electricity also. Yogis call it *prana* — the inner bio-energy or bio-electricity. Through sound that can be changed immediately.

That's why, when listening to classical music, you feel a certain silence surrounding you: your inner body energy is changed. Listen to a madman and you will feel you are also going crazy: because the madman is in a chaos of body electricity and his words and sounds carry that electricity to you. Sit with an enlightened person and suddenly you feel everything within you is falling in a rhythm. Suddenly you feel a different quality of energy arising in you.

That's why Patanjali says the repetition of Aum and meditation on it destroys all obstacles. What are the obstacles? Now he describes each obstacle, and how they can be destroyed by repeating the sound of Aum and meditating on it; we will have to ponder over.

*Disease, languor, doubt, carelessness, laziness, sensuality, delusion, impotency and instability are the obstacles that distract the mind.*

Take each: disease. For Patanjali, disease means disease. It is a non-rhythmic way of your inner bio-energy.
You feel uncomfortable. If this uncomfort, this dis-ease,
continues, sooner or later it will affect your body.
Patanjali will agree with acupuncture absolutely, and in
Soviet Russia a man named Kirlian will agree with
Patanjali absolutely. All the three trends. . . Acupuncture is not concerned with enlightenment, but acupuncture is concerned how the body becomes diseased,
how illness happens, and acupuncture has discovered
seven hundred points on the body where the inner bio-
energy touches the physical body — touchpoints — seven
hundred all around the body.

Whenever the electricity is not flowing in a circle in
these seven hundred points — some gaps are there, few
points are no more functioning, through few points the
electricity is no more moving, blocks are there, electricity is cut, it is not a circle — then disease happens. So
acupuncture believes that without any medicine, without any other treatment, if you allow the bio-energy
flow to become a circle, the disease disappears. And for
five thousand years. . .acupuncture was born almost
when Patanjali was alive.

As I told you, that after two thousand five hundred
years there comes a peak of human consciousness. It
happened in the time of Buddha; in China Lao Tzu,
Chuang Tzu, Confucius; in India Buddha, Mahavira
and others; in Greece Heraclitus; in Iran Zoroaster: the
peak phenomenon happened. All the religions that you
see now in the world derive from that moment of human consciousness. From that peak, the Himalaya, all
the rivers of all the religions have been flowing for these
two thousand five hundred years.

Just the same, two thousand five hundred years
before Buddha there was a peak phenomenon. Patanjali, Rishabh — the originator of Jainism — the Vedas,
Upanishads, acupuncture in China, yoga in India and
tantra: these all happened. They attained a peak. Never

again that peak has been surpassed. And from that very remote past, five thousand years back, yoga, tantra, acupuncture, they have been flowing like rivers.

And there is a certain phenomenon which Jung called "synchronicity". When a certain principle is born, not only one person becomes aware of it—many on the earth, as if the whole earth is ready to receive it. Einstein is reported to have said that "If I had not discovered the theory of relativity, then within a year somebody else would have discovered it." Why? Because many people all over the earth were working in the same direction.

When Darwin discovered the theory of evolution, that man has evolved out of monkeys, that there is a constant struggle for the survival of the fittest, another man—Wallace Russell—discovered it. He was in Philippines, and both were friends. But for many years they had not known each other. Darwin was working for twenty years continuously, but he was a lazy man. He has many fragments and everything was ready, but he will not make a book out of it and he will not present it to the scientific society of those days.

Friends again and again will request that "Do it. Otherwise somebody else will do it." And then one day, from Philippines, a letter arrived and the whole theory was presented in that letter by Russell. And he was a friend, but they both were working separately. They never knew that both are working on the same. And then he became afraid, what to do? Because he will become the discoverer, and for twenty years he had known the principle. He rushed, somehow managed to write a report, presented it to the scientific society.

After three months, everybody else became aware that Russell has also discovered. Russell was really a very beautiful person. He declared that the discovery goes to Darwin because for twenty years, whether he has presented it or not. . . But he is the discoverer.

And this is happening many times. Suddenly a thought becomes very prominent, as if a thought is trying to take a womb somewhere. And as is the way of the nature, it never takes risks. One man may miss; then many men have to be tried. Nature never takes risks! A tree will drop millions of seeds. One seed may miss, may not fall on the right ground, may be destroyed, but millions of seeds — there is no possibility all the seeds will be destroyed.

When you make love, in one ejaculation millions of seeds are thrown by the man — one of them will reach to the egg of the woman — but millions. Almost in one ejaculation, a man releases as many seeds as there are men on the earth right now. One man in one ejaculation can give birth to the whole earth, to the whole population of the earth. Nature takes no risks. It tries many ways. One may miss, two may miss, a million may miss, but with millions at least one will reach and become alive.

Jung discovered a principle which he calls "synchronicity". It is a rare thing. We know one principle of cause and effect: a cause produces an effect. Synchronicity says whenever something happens, parallel to it many things similar happen. Yet we don't know why it happens, because it is not a cause and effect phenomenon. They are not related with each other as cause and effect.

How can you relate Buddha and Heraclitus? But the same principle. Buddha never heard of Heraclitus; Heraclitus we cannot imagine ever knew about Buddha. They lived in separate worlds. There was no communication. But the same principle of flow, of river-like existence, of momentary existence both gave to the world. They are not causing each other. They are parallel. A synchronicity exists as if the whole existence at that moment wants to produce a certain principle and wants to make it manifest — it manifested, and it will not depend only on Buddha or only on Heraclitus: many it will try. And there were others also who went into oblivion: they were not so prominent. Buddha and

Heraclitus became the most prominent. They were the most forceful Masters.

In the days of Patanjali, a principle was born. You can call it the principle of *prana* — bio-energy. In China it took the form of acupuncture, in India it took the form of the whole system of yoga. How it happens when the body energy is not flowing rightly you feel uncomfort? Because a gap exists in you, an absence, and you feel something is missing. This is dis-ease in the beginning. First it will be felt in the mind. As I told you, first it will be felt in the unconscious.

You may not be aware of it; in your dreams it will come first; in your dreams you will see illness, disease, somebody dying, something wrong. A nightmare will happen in your unconscious because the unconscious is nearest to the body and nearest to nature. From the unconscious it will come up to the subconscious; then you will feel irritated. You will feel that stars are wrong, whatsoever you do goes wrong. You would like to love a person, and you try to love but you cannot love. You would like to help somebody, but you only hinder. Everything goes wrong.

You think some bad influence, some star in the high sky — no — something in the subconscious, some uncomfort, and you get irritated, angry, and the cause is somewhere in the unconscious. You are finding the cause somewhere else. Then the cause comes to the conscious. Then you start feeling that you are ill, and then it moves to the body. It has been always moving to the body, and suddenly you feel ill.

In Soviet Russia a photographer, a rare scientist, Kirlian, has discovered that before one person becomes ill, six months before, the illness can be photographed. And this is going to be one of the greatest discoveries in the world of twentieth century. It will transform the whole concept of man, disease, medicine, everything. It is a revolutionary concept, and he has been working thirty years and he has almost proved everything scientifically that when a disease comes to the body, first it comes to the electric aura around the body. A gap comes to the. . .

You may be going to have a tumor in the stomach after six months. Right now no base exists. No scientist can find anything wrong with your stomach; everything is okay, no problem. You can be checked thoroughly and you are right. But Kirlian photographs the body on a very sensitive plate: he has developed the most sensitive plates. And on that plate not only your body is photographed, but around the body a light aura which you carry always. And in that aura, near the stomach there is a hole in the aura — not exactly in the physical body, but something is disturbed.

And now he says that he can predict that within six months there will be a tumor. And after six months, when the tumor comes to the body, x-rays show the same picture as he had taken six months before. So Kirlian says without being ill it can be predicted — and it can be cured before ever it comes to the body, if the body aura becomes more circulating. He doesn't know how it can be cured; acupuncture knows, Patanjali knows how it can be cured.

Disease for Patanjali is some disturbance in the body aura, in the *prana*, in the bio-energy, in the electricity of your body. That's why through Aum it can be cured. Sometime, you sit lonely in a temple. Go through some old temple where nobody goes, under the dome — circular dome is just to reflect the sound — so sit under it, chant Aum loudly and meditate on it. And let the sound reflect back and fall upon you like a rain, and suddenly you will feel after a few minutes your whole body is getting peaceful, calm, quiet: the body energy is getting settled.

The first thing is disease. And if you are ill in your *prana* energy, you cannot go far. How can you go far with illness hanging around you like a cloud? You cannot enter into deeper realms. A certain health is needed.

The Indian word for health is very meaningful: it is *swasthya*. The very word means "to be oneself". The word for health in Sanskrit means to be oneself, to be centered. The English word health is also beautiful. It comes from the same word, the same root, from where holy and whole come. When you are whole you are healthy and when you are whole you are holy also.

It is always good to go to the roots of words because they arose of a long experience of humanity. Words have not come accidentally. When a person feels whole, his body energy is running in a circle. The circle is the most perfect thing in the world. A perfect circle is a symbol of God. Energy is not being wasted. It circulates again and again; it goes on moving like a wheel; it perpetuates itself.

When you are whole you are healthy, and when you are healthy you are holy also, because that holy word also comes from whole. A perfectly healthy person is holy, but then there will be problems. If you go to the monasteries you will find there all types of ill people. In fact, ill people only go there. A healthy person you will ask what he has to do in a monastery. Ill people go there, abnormal people go there. Something is basically wrong with them. That's why they escape from the world and go there.

Patanjali makes it a first rule that you should be healthy, because if you are not healthy you cannot go far. Your illness, your discomfort, your inner broken circle of energy, will be a stone on your neck. When you will meditate you will feel ill at ease. When you would like to pray, you cannot pray, you would like to rest. A low energy level will be there. And with low energy how can you go far? And to reach to God? And for Patanjali God is the farthest point: much energy is needed. A healthy body, a healthy mind, a healthy being is needed. Disease is dis-ease — dis-ease in the body energy. Aum will help and other things also we will discuss. But here Patanjali is talking about how Aum, the sound itself, helps you inside to become a whole.

For Patanjali, and for many others who have searched deeply into human energy, one fact has become very certain—you must know about it—and that is, the more you are ill, the more sensual. When you are perfectly healthy you are not sensual. Ordinarily, we think just the contrary—that a healthy man has to be sensual, sexual, this and that: he has to enjoy the world and the body. It is not the case. When you are ill, then more sensuality, more sex, grips you. When you are perfectly healthy, sex and sensuality disappear.

Why it happens? Because when you are perfectly healthy you are so happy with yourself you don't need the other. When you are ill, you are so unhappy with yourself you need the other. And this is the paradox: when you are ill you need the other, and the other also needs you when she or he is ill. And two ill persons meeting, the illness is not doubled, it is multiplied.

That's what happens in a marriage: two ill persons meeting multiply illnesses and then the whole thing becomes ugly and a hell. Ill persons need others, and they are precisely the persons who will create trouble when they are related. A healthy person doesn't need. But if a healthy person loves, it is not a need, it is a sharing. The whole phenomenon changes. He is not in need of anybody. He has so much that he can share.

Ill person needs sex, a healthy person loves, and love is a totally different thing. And when two healthy persons meet, health is multiplied. Then they can become helpers to each other for the ultimate. They can go together for the ultimate, helping each other. But the need disappears. It is no more a need, it is no more a dependence.

Whenever you have an uncomfortable feeling with yourself, don't try to drown it into sex and sensuality.

Rather, try to become more healthy. *Yogasanas* will help. We will discuss about them later on when Patanjali talks about them. Right now, he says, if you chant Aum and meditate on it, disease will disappear. And he is right! Not only the disease that is there will disappear, but the disease that was to come in the future, that will also disappear!

If a man can become a perfect chanting so that the chanter is completely lost — only a pure consciousness, a flame of light and all around, chanting — the energy falls into a circle, becomes a circle. And then you have one of the most euphoric moments in life. When the energy falls into a circle, becomes a harmony, there is no discord, no conflict, you have become one. But ordinarily also, disease will be a hindrance. If you are ill, you need treatment.

Patanjali's yoga system and Hindu system of medicine, Ayurveda, developed simultaneously, together. Ayurveda is totally different than allopathy. Allopathy is suppressive of the disease. Allopathy has developed side by side with Christianity; it is a byproduct. And because Christianity is suppressive, allopathy is suppressive. If you are ill, allopathy immediately suppresses the illness. Then the illness tries some other weak point to come up. Then from somewhere else it explodes. Then you suppress it from there, then from somewhere else it explodes. But with allopathy, you go on from one illness to another, from another to another, but it is never-ending process.

Ayurveda has a totally different concept. Illness should not be suppressed: it should be released. A catharsis is needed. So Ayurvedic medicine is given to the ill person so that the illness comes up and is thrown out, a catharsis. So the beginning doses of Ayurvedic medicine may make you more ill, and it takes a long time because it is not a suppression. It cannot be done right now: it is a long process. The illness has to be thrown, and your inner energy has to become a harmony so the health comes from within. The medicine will throw the illness out, and the healing force will replace it from your own being.

They developed Ayurveda and yoga together. If you are doing *yogasanas*, if you are following Patanjali, then never go to an allopathic doctor. If you are not following Patanjali, then there is no problem. But if you are following the yoga system and working many things in your body energy, then never go to allopathy because they are contrary. Then seek an ayurvedic doctor or homeopathy or naturopathy — anything that helps catharsis.

But if there is a disease, first tackle it. Don't move with the disease. With my methods it is very easy to get rid of a disease. Because Patanjali's method of Aum, of chanting and meditating, is a very mild one. But in those days, that was enough strong because people were simple, they lived with nature. Illness was rare; health was common. Now just the opposite is the case: health is rare, illness is common, and people are very complex, they don't live near the nature.

There was a survey in London. One million boys and girls have not seen a cow. They have seen only pictures of a cow. By and by, we are bracketed into a manmade world; concrete buildings, asphalt roads — all manmade — technology, big machinery, cars. Nature is thrown somewhere into the dark, and nature is a healing force. And then man becomes more and more complex. He doesn't listen to his nature; he listens to the demands of the civilization, demands of the society. He completely is out of contact with his own inner being.

Then Patanjali's mild methods won't help much. Hence, my dynamic, chaotic methods — because you are almost mad, you need mad methods which can bring out all that is suppressed within you and throw it out. But health is a must. One who goes for a long journey must see that he is healthy. Ill, bedridden, it is difficult to move.

Second obstacle is languor: languor means a man who has very low energy search. He wants to seek and search, but a very low energy search—lukewarm. He wants to evaporate, but that's not possible. Such a man always talks about God, *moksha*, yoga, this and that, but talks. With low energy level you can talk; that's all you can do. If you want to do something, you need a high energy effort.

Once it happened: Mulla went with his horse and buggy to some town. It was a hot summer day; Mulla was perspiring. Suddenly, on the road, the horse stopped, looked back at Mulla and said, "Saints alive, but it is too hot!" Mulla could not believe. He thought he has gone crazy because of the heat, because how the horse can say? How the horse can talk?

So he looked around if anybody else has heard, but there was nobody except his dog who was sitting in the buggy. Not finding anyone, but just to get rid of the idea, he told to the dog, "Have you heard what he says?" The dog says, "Oh, he is just like anybody else—always talking about the weather and doing nothing."

This is the man of languor—always talking about God, doing nothing. He always talks of great things, and this talk is just to hide a wound. He talks so that he can forget that he is not doing anything about it. Through a cloud of talk, he escapes. Talking again and again about it, he thinks he is doing something, but talk is not a doing. You can go on talking about the weather, you can go on talking about God. And if you don't do anything, you are simply wasting your energy.

This type of person can become a minister, a priest, a pundit. These are low-energy people. And they can become very proficient in talking—so proficient that they can deceive, because they always talk about beautiful and great things. Others listen to them and get deceived; philosophers—these are all people of languor. Patanjali is not a philosopher. He himself is a scientist, and he wants others to be scientists. Much effort is needed.

Through the chanting of Aum and meditating on it, your low energy level will become high. How it happens? Why you are on a low energy level always, always feeling exhausted, tired? Even in the morning when you get up, you are tired. What is happening to you? Somewhere in your system there are leakages; you leak energy. You are not aware, but you are like a bucket with holes. Every day you fill the bucket, but you see it is always empty, getting empty. This leakage has to be stopped.

How energy leaks through the body? These are deep problems for bio-energetics. The body leaks always from fingers of the hand, of the feet, eyes. The energy cannot leak through the head: it is round. Anything round helps the body to preserve. That's why yoga postures—*siddhasana*, *padmasana*—they make the whole body round.

A person who is sitting in a *siddhasana* puts his both hands together because the body energy leaks through the fingers. When both the hands are put together on top of each other, the energy moves from one hand into the other. It becomes a circle. Feet, legs, are also put on each other so that the energy moves in your own body and doesn't leak.

Eyes are closed because eyes release almost eighty percent of your bio-energy. That's why, if you continuously are traveling and you go on looking out of the train or the car, you will feel so tired. If you travel with closed eyes, you will not feel so tired. And you go on looking at unnecessary things, even reading advertisements on the walls. You use your eyes too much, and when eyes are tired the whole body is tired. Eyes give the indication that now it is enough.

A yogi tries to remain with closed eyes as much as possible, with hands and legs crossing each other, so the energy moves into each other. He sits with the spine straight. If the spine is straight while you are sitting, you will preserve more energy than any other way – because when the spine is straight, the gravitation of the earth cannot force much energy out of you, because it touches only one point of the spine. That's why when you are sitting in such a leaning posture, slanting, you think you are resting. But Patanjali says you are leaking energy, because more of your body is under the influence of gravitation.

This won't help. Straight spine, with closed hands and legs, with closed eyes, you have become a circle: that circle is represented by Shivalinga. You must have seen the Shivalinga – the phallic symbol, as it is known in the West. In fact, it is the inner bio-energy circle, just egg shaped.

When your body energy flows rightly, it becomes like an egg: the shape is like an egg, exactly like an egg. And that is symbolized in the Shivalinga. You become a Shiva. When the energy is flowing into yourself again and again, not moving out, then languor disappears. It will not disappear by talking; it will not disappear by reading scriptures; it will not disappear by philosophizing. It will disappear only when your energy is not leaking.

Try to preserve it. The more you preserve, the better. But in the West, something just the opposite is being taught – that it is good to release energy through sex, this and that – release energy. It is good if you are not using it in any other way; otherwise you will get mad. And whenever there is too much energy, it is better to release it through sex. Sex is the simplest method to release it.

But it can be used, can be made creative! It can give you a rebirth, a resurrection. You can know millions of euphoric stages through it; you can rise higher and higher through it. It is the ladder to reach the God. If you go on every day releasing it, you will never have such built up energy that you can take even the first step towards the divine. Preserve!

Patanjali is against sex, and that is the difference between Patanjali and tantra. Tantra uses sex as a method; Patanjali wants you to bypass it. And there are persons, almost fifty percent, to whom tantra will suit; and fifty percent to whom yoga will suit. One has to find what will suit him. Both can be used, and through both, people reach. And neither is wrong or right. It depends on you. One will be right for you and one wrong for you, but remember, for you! It is not an absolute categorical statement.

Something may be right for you and wrong for somebody else. And both the systems were born together, tantra and yoga — twin systems, exactly at the same time — this is the synchronicity. As if man and woman need each other, tantra and yoga need each other; they become a complete thing. If there is only yoga, then only fifty percent can reach; fifty percent will be in trouble. If there is only tantra, then fifty percent can reach; the other fifty percent will be in trouble. And this has happened.

And sometimes, not knowing where you are moving, what you are doing, if you go on without a Master, not knowing who you are and what will suit you. . . You may be a woman and just dressed like a man, and you think yourself a man — then you will be in trouble. You may be a man and dressed like a woman, and you think yourself a woman — you will be in trouble.

Trouble arises whenever you don't understand who you are. A Master is needed to give you clear-cut direction that this is for you. So remember; whenever I say something, that this is for you, don't go on spreading to others, because it has been specifically told to you. People are curious. If you tell them, they will try. It may not be for them. It may be harmful even. And remember, if it is not helpful, it is going to be harmful. There is no in-between. Something is either helpful for you or harmful.

Languor is one of the greatest obstacles, but it disappears through the chanting of Aum. The Aum creates within you the Shivalinga, the egg-shaped energy circle. When you become perceptive you can even see it. With your closed eyes if you chant Aum for few months, meditate, you can see within you, your body has disappeared. There will be just a bio-energy, an electric phenomenon, and the shape will be the Shivalinga shape.

The moment this happens to you, languor has disappeared. Now you are a high energy. Now you can move mountains. Now you will feel talk is not enough; something has to be done. And the energy level is so high that something can be done now. People come to me and they ask me what to do, but I look at them and I see that they are leaking energy; they cannot do anything. The first thing is to drop this leakage. Only when you have energy, then ask what can be done.

"Doubt" — Sanskrit has many words for doubt; English has only one word. So try to understand; I will explain you. There is a doubt against trust. In Sanskrit it is called *shanka* — doubt against trust, one pair. Then there is a doubt called *sanshaya* — Patanjali is talking about *sanshaya* now — doubt against certainty, against decisiveness. A man of uncertainty, a man who is not decisive, he is in *sanshaya* — in doubt. This is not against trust because trust is to trust in somebody. This is against self-confidence; you don't trust in yourself. That's a different thing.

So whatsoever you do, you are not certain whether you want to do it or don't want to do it, whether it will be good to go into it or not — an indecisiveness. With an indecisive mind, you cannot enter on the path — not on the path of Patanjali. You have to be decisive! You have to take a decision! Difficult it is because a part of you always goes on saying no. Then how to take the decision? Think about as much as you can; give it as much time as you can. Think all the possibilities, all the alternatives, and then decide. And once you decide, then drop all doubting.

Before that, use it: do whatsoever you can do with the doubt. Think all the possibilities and then choose. Of course it is not going to be a total decision; in the beginning it is not possible. It will be a major decision — majority of your mind will say yes. Once you decide, then never doubt. The doubt will raise its head. You simply say, "I have decided! — finished! It is not a total decision; all doubts are not discarded. But whatsoever could be done, I have done. I have thought it out as completely as it was possible and I have chosen."

Once you choose then never give doubt again any cooperation, because doubt exists in you through your cooperation. You go on giving energy to it, and again and again you start thinking about it. Then an indecisiveness is created. Indecisiveness is a very bad state of affairs — you are in a very bad shape. If you cannot decide anything, how can you do? How can you act?

How Aum — the sound and the meditation — will help? It helps, because once you become silent, peaceful, decision becomes easier. Then you are no more a crowd, not a chaos: many voices talking together and you don't know which voice is yours. Aum, the chanting, the meditating on it — voices become silent. Many voices — now you can see they are not yours. Your mother is speaking, your father is speaking, your brothers, your teachers, they are not yours. You can discard them easily because they don't need any attention.

When you become silent under the chanting of Aum, you are sheltered, calm, quiet, collected. In that collectedness you can see which is the real voice which is coming from you, which is authentic. It is as if you are standing in a marketplace, and many people are talking and many things are going on, and you cannot decide what is happening. In a share-market, people are shouting — they know their language — you cannot understand what is happening, whether they have gone mad or not.

Then you move to a Himalayan retreat. You sit in a cave, you simply chant. You simply calm down yourself, all nervousness disappears, you become one, collected. In that moment, decisiveness is possible. And then decide, and then don't look back. Then forget! — it is decided and decided. Now there is no going back. Then go ahead.

Sometimes the doubt will follow, bark at you just like a dog. But if you don't listen, don't pay attention, by and by it stops. Give it a chance, think all that is possible, and once decided, drop it, and *Aumkar* will help you to come to a decisiveness. Here, doubt means indecisiveness, carelessness. The Sanskrit word is *pramad*. The *pramad* means as if one is walking in sleep. Carelessness is part of it; exact translation will be, "Don't be a zombie: don't walk in hypnosis."

But you live in hypnosis not knowing it at all. The whole society is trying to hypnotize you for certain things, and that creates *pramad:* that creates a sleepiness in you. What is happening? You are not aware, otherwise you will be simply surprised what is happening. It is so familiar. That's why you don't become aware. You are being pulled by many manipulators, and their method of manipulating you is creating hypnosis in you.

For example, on every radio, on every TV screen, on every film, on every newspaper, magazine, they go on advertising for a certain thing — "Lux toilet soap". You think you are not affected, but every day you hear, "Lux toilet soap, Lux toilet soap, Lux toilet soap". It is a chanting. In the night, on the streets, neon lights say "Lux toilet soap". And now they have found it out that if you flicker the light it is more impressive. If it goes on and off, then it is even more impressive because then you have to read it again: "Lux toilet soap". Then the light goes on, comes again, and you have to read it again: "Lux toilet soap".

You are chanting Aum! It is going deeper in your subconscious. You think you are not bothered, you think you are not befooled by these people — all these beautiful naked women standing near Lux toilet soap and saying, "Why I am beautiful? Why my face is so beautiful? Because of Lux toilet soap." You know that you are not, but you are affected. Suddenly, one day you go to the market, go to the shop, and you ask for a Lux toilet soap. The shopkeeper asks, "Which soap?" Then suddenly it bubbles up: "Lux toilet soap".

You are being hypnotized by the businessmen, political leaders, educationists, priests, because everybody has an investment in you if you are hypnotized. Then you can be used. The politicians go on saying that "This is your mother country, and if the mother country is in difficulty, go to the war: become a martyr."

What nonsense! The whole earth is your mother. Is earth divided into India, Pakistan, Germany, England, or is it one? But the politicians are continuously hammering your mind that only this part of the earth is your mother; you have to save it. Even if your life is lost, it is very good. And they go on: devotion to the country, nationalism, patriotism — all nonsense terms, but if they are hammered continuously, you become hypnotized. Then you can sacrifice yourself.

You are sacrificing your life in a hypnosis because of slogans. A flag, an ordinary piece of cloth, becomes so important through hypnosis. This is "our national flag" — millions can die for it. If there are beings on other planets and they look sometimes at the earth, they will think, "These people are simply mad." For a cloth — a piece of cloth — because you have insulted "our flag", and this cannot be tolerated. . .

Then religions go on preaching: you are a Christian, a Hindu, a Mohammedan, this and that, and they make you feel that you are a Christian, and then you are on a crusade: "Kill others who are not Christians. This is your duty!" And they teach you such absurd things, but you still believe because they go on saying it. Adolf Hitler says in his autobiography, "Mein Kampf", that if you repeat a lie continuously it becomes a truth. And he knows. Nobody knows as well as he knows because he repeated himself and created the phenomenon.

*Pramad* means a state of hypnosis, manipulated, moving sleepily. Then carelessness is bound to come because you are not yourself. Then you do everything without any care. You move and stumble on. In relationship with things, with persons, you continuously are stumbling; you are not going anywhere, you are just like a drunkard. But everybody else is just like you, so you don't have the opportunity to feel that you are a drunkard.

Be careful. How Aum will help you to be careful? It will drop hypnosis. In fact, if you simply chant Aum without meditating, it will also become a hypnosis: that is the difference between the ordinary chanting of a mantra and Patanjali's way. Chant it and remain aware.

If you chant Aum and remain aware, this Aum and its chanting will become a dehypnotizing force. It will destroy all the hypnosis that exists around you, that has been created in you by the society and the manipulators, politicians. It will be a dehypnotization.

Once it was asked in America, somebody asked Vivekananda that "What is the difference between ordinary hypnosis and your chanting of Aum?" He said, "Chanting of Aum is a dehypnosis: it is moving in the reverse gear." The process seems to be the same, but the gear is reverse. And how it becomes reverse? If you are meditating also, then by and by you become so silent and so aware, so careful, that nobody can hypnotize you. Now you are beyond the reach of priests and politicians — the prisoners. Now, for the first time, you are an individual, and then you become careful. Then you move with care, each step with care because millions are the pitfalls all around you.

"Laziness" — *alasya:* there is much laziness accumulated in you. It comes for certain reasons — because you don't see the point of doing anything. And even if you do, nothing is achieved. If you don't do, nothing is lost. Then a laziness settles in the heart. Laziness means simply that you have lost the zest for life.

Children are not lazy. They are bubbling with energy. You have to force them to go to sleep; you have to force them to be silent; you have to force them to sit for few minutes in order to relax. They are not tense: this is your idea. They are full of energy — such tiny beings with so much energy! From where this energy comes? They are still unfrustrated. They don't know that in this life, whatsoever you do nothing is achieved. They are unaware — blissfully unaware: that's why so much energy.

And you have been doing many things, and nothing is achieved — laziness settles. It is like dust settling in you — of all failures, frustrations, every dream gone sour. It settles! Then you become lazy. In the morning, you think, "For what to get up again? For what!" There is no answer. You have to get up because somehow bread is to be earned. And there is a wife, and there are children, and you are caught in the trap. You move to the office somehow; you come back somehow. There is no zest! You drag! You are not happy doing anything.

How the chanting of Aum and meditating on it will help it? It helps! — certainly helps, because when for the first time you chant Aum and watch and meditate, the first effort in your life seems to bring a fulfillment. You feel so happy chanting it, you feel so blissful chanting it, that the first effort has succeeded.

Now a new zest arises. The dust is being thrown. A new courage, a new confidence is attained. Now you think you also can do something, you can also achieve something. Everything is not a failure. Maybe the outward journey is a failure, but the inward journey is not a failure. Even the first step brings so many flowers. Now hope arises; confidence settles again. You are again a child — of the inner world. . .a new birth. You can again laugh, run, play. Again you are born.

This is what Hindus call the twice-born. This is the next birth, a second birth. The first birth was in the outside world. It has proved a failure; that's why you feel so lethargic. And by the time one is forty, one starts thinking of death — how to die, how to be finished.

If people don't commit suicide, it is not that they are happy. It is only simply because they don't see even any hope even in death. Even death seems to be hopeless. It is not because they love life that they are not committing suicide — no! They are so frustrated that they know that even death is not going to give anything. So why commit unnecessarily? Why take the trouble? So go on as things are.

"Sensuality": why you feel sensual, sexual? You feel sexual because you accumulate energy, unused energy, and you don't know what to do with it. So, naturally, at the first center of sex, it accumulates. And you don't know any other centers, and you don't know how it can flow upwards.

It is like you have got an airplane, but you don't know what it is so you search into it, and then you think, "It has wheels, so must be a sort of vehicle." So you yoke horses to it and use it as a bullock cart. It can be used! Then someday, by accident, you discover that bullocks are not needed. It has a certain engine in it, so you use it as a motor car. Then you go deeper and deeper in search. Then you wonder why these wings? Then one day you use it as it should be used — as an airplane.

When you move inside you, you discover many things. But if you don't move, then there is only sexuality. You gather energy, then what to do with it? You don't know anything that you can fly upwards. You become a bullock cart: sex is behaving like a bullock cart. You gather energy. You eat food, you drink water, energy is created, energy is there; if you don't use it, you will go mad. Then the energy goes round and round within you. It makes you crazy. You have to do something. If you don't do something, you will go crazy; you will explode. Sex is the easiest safety valve — energy moves back into nature.

This is foolish because the energy comes from the nature. You eat food: it is eating nature. You drink water; it is drinking nature. You take a sunbath; it is eating sun. Continuously, you are eating nature, and then you throw it out back to the nature. The whole thing seems to be baseless, useless, with no meaning. What is the use of it? Then you become lethargic.

The energy must go higher. You must become a transformer: through you nature must become supernature; only then there is meaning, significance. Through you matter must become mind; mind must become supermind. Through you nature must reach to the supernature: the lowest must become the highest. Only then there is a significance — a felt significance.

Then your life has a deep, deep significance. You are not worthless; you are not like dirt. You are a god! When you have moved through you the nature to the supernature, you have become a god. Patanjali is a god. You become a Master of Masters.

But, ordinarily, sensuality means that energy gathers, and you have to throw it out. You don't know what to do with it. First you gather it: first you go on seeking for food, doing much effort to earn bread. Then you absorb the bread and create energy, because sex energy is the most refined energy in your body, the most refined! And then you throw it out, and then you again go in the circle.

It is a vicious circle. When you throw it out, the body needs energy. You eat, collect, throw: how can you feel that you have some meaning? You seem to be in a rut leading nowhere. How Aum will help? How meditating on it will help? Once you start meditating on Aum, other centers start functioning.

When the energy flows, inside you becomes a circle. Then sex center is not the only center which is functioning. Your whole body becomes a circle. From the sex center it rises to the second, to the third, fourth, fifth, seventh center; then again sixth, fifth, fourth, third, second, first. It becomes an inner circle and it passes other centers.

Just because energy is accumulated, it rises high: the level of energy goes high, just like a dam: the water goes on coming from the river, and the dam is not allowing it to go out. The water rises high, and other centers, other chakras in your body, start opening—because when the energy flows, they become dynamic forces, dynamos. They start functioning.

It is as if a waterfall and a dynamo start functioning; the waterfall is dry and the dynamo cannot start. When the energy flows upwards, your highest chakras start working, functioning. This is how Aum helps. It makes you calm, collected, one. Energy rises high; sensuality disappears. Sex becomes meaningless, childish, not yet gone, but becomes childish. You don't feel sensual; you don't have an urge for it.

It is still there. If you are not careful, it will take your grip again. You can fall, because this is not the ultimate happening. You are not yet crystalized but a glimpse has happened that the energy can give you inner ecstatic states. And sex is the lowest ecstasy. Higher ecstasies are possible. When the higher becomes possible, the lower disappears automatically. You need not renounce it. If you renounce, then your energy is not moving high. If the energy is moving high, there is no need to renounce. It simply becomes useless. It simply drops by itself. Non-functioning it becomes delusion.

As you are, psychoanalysts say that if you stop

dreaming you will go mad. Dreams are needed because in your state of mind delusions are needed. Delusions, deceptions, illusions, dreams are needed because you are sleepy, and in sleep, dreams are a necessity.

They have been experimenting in America, that if you are not allowed for seven days to dream, immediately you start a delusion trip: with open eyes you start seeing things which are not. You start talking to persons which are not, you start seeing visions. You are mad. Just seven days no dreaming, and you become delusionary. Hallucinations start happening. Your dreams are a catharsis—an inbuilt catharsis, so every night you delude yourself. By the morning you are a little sober, but by the evening again you have gathered much energy. In the night you have to dream and throw it out.

This happens to drivers, and many accidents happen because of this. In the night, accidents happen near about four, four o'clock in the morning, because the driver has been driving the whole night. He has not been dreaming; now the dream energy accumulates. And with open eyes he is driving and he starts seeing illusions. "The road is straight," he says. "There is nobody: no truck is coming." With open eyes he goes into a truck. Or he sees a truck coming, and just to avoid it—and there was no truck—just to avoid it, he crashes against a tree.

Much research has been done why so many accidents happen nearabout four. In fact, nearabout four you dream too much. Four to five, six, you dream too much! That is dream time. You have slept well; now there is no need for sleep, you can dream. In the morning you dream, and that time if you don't dream, are not allowed to dream you will create delusions. You will dream with open eyes.

Delusion means dreaming with open eyes, but everybody is dreaming that way. You see a woman and you think she is absolutely beautiful. That may not be the case. You may be projecting an illusion on her. You may be sexually starved. Then energy is there and you delude. After two days, three days, the woman looks ordinary. You think you have been deceived. Nobody is deceiving you; you yourself. . . But you deluded. Lovers delude each other. They dream with open eyes and then they are frustrated. Nobody is at fault, just your state.

Patanjali says delusion will disappear if you chant Aum with mindfulness. How it will happen?—because delusion means a dreaming state, when you are lost. You are no more there: just the dream is there. If you meditate on Aum, you have created the sound of Aum and you are a witness, you are there! Your presence cannot allow any dream to happen! Whenever you are, there is no dream. Whenever there is a dream, you are not. You both cannot be together. If you are there, the dream will disappear. Or, you will have to disappear. Both together cannot be. Dream and awareness never meet. That's why delusion disappears by witnessing the sound of Aum.

"Impotency": impotency is also there, continuously felt. You feel yourself helpless: that is impotency. You feel you cannot do anything, you are worthless, of no use. You may pretend that you are somebody, but your pretension also shows that deep down you feel the no-bodiness. You may pretend that you are very powerful, but your pretension is nothing but hiding.

Mulla Nasruddin entered a tavern with a sheet of paper in his hand and declared, "Here are the names of the people I can lick,"—hundred names. One man stood up: he was a tiny man; Mulla could have licked him. But he had two pistols around his belt. He came near with a pistol in his hand and he said, "Is my name also there?"

Mulla looked at him and said, "Yes." The man said, "You cannot lick me." Mulla said, "Are you sure?" The man said, "Absolutely sure. Look!" And he showed the pistol. Mulla said, "Then okay. I will cut your name out of the list."

You can pretend that you are very powerful, but whenever you come in an encounter you start feeling the helplessness and the powerlessness. Man is impotent because only the whole can be potent—not man. The part cannot be potent. Only God is potent; man is impotent.

When you chant *Aumkar*, Aum, for the first time you feel that you are no more an island. You become one part of the whole universal sound. For the first time you feel yourself potent, but now this potency need not be violent, need not be aggressive. In fact, a powerful man is never aggressive. Only impotent people become aggressive to prove themselves—that we are powerful.

. . .*and instability are the obstacles that distract the mind:* you start one thing and then stop—on and off— you start again and then off. Nothing is possible with this instability. One has to persevere, to go on digging the hole at the same spot continuously. If you leave your effort, your mind is such after few days you will have to start from the ABC again; it rewinds itself, it unwinds itself. You do something for few days, then you leave. You will be thrown back to your first day of doing—again ABC. Then you can do much without achieving anything. Aum will give you a taste.

Why you start and stop? People come to me and they say they meditated for one year, then they stopped. And I ask them, "How you were feeling?" They say, "Very, very good we were feeling"—but then why you stopped? Nobody stops when somebody is feeling very, very good. And they say "We were very happy and then we stopped."—it is impossible. If you were happy, how can you stop? Then they say, "Not exactly happy."

But they are in trouble. They pretend even that they are happy. If you are happy in a certain thing, you continue. You stop only when it is a boring thing, a boredom, unhappiness. With Aum, Patanjali says, you will feel the first taste of dropping into the universal. That taste will become your happiness and instability will go. That's why he says chanting Aum and witnessing it all obstacles drop.

*Anguish, despair, tremors and irregular*
*breathing are the symptoms of a distracted*
*mind.*

These are the symptoms. Anguish: always anxiety-ridden, always split, always an anxious mind, always sad, in despair, subtle tremors in the body energy, because when the body energy is not running in a circle you have subtle tremors, a trembling, fear and irregular breathing. Then your breathing cannot be rhythmic. It cannot be a song; it cannot be a harmony. An irregular breathing. . .

These are the symptoms of a distracted mind, and against these are the symptoms of a mind who is centered. The chanting of Aum will make you centered. Your breathing will become rhythmic. Your tremors in the body will disappear; you will not be nervous. Sadness will be replaced by a happy feeling, a joy, a subtle blissfulness on your face, for no reason at all. Simply happy you are: just being here you are happy; just breathing you are happy. You don't demand much, and instead of anguish there will be bliss.

*To remove these, meditate on one principle.*

These symptoms of a distracted mind can be removed by meditating on one principle. That one principle is *pranava*—Aum, the universal sound.

# From

# Chaos

# To

# Chaos

# With

# Aum

The first question:

*The way seems to be towards peace and awareness. Why then is everyone and everything around you in such a chaos?*

**B**ECAUSE I AM A CHAOS! And only out of a chaos a cosmos is born; there is no other way. You are like old, very old, ancient buildings; you cannot be renovated. For millions of lives you have been here. First you have to be demolished completely, and only then recreated.

Renovation is possible, but that won't help long. It will be just a surface decoration. Deep in your foundations you will remain the old, and the whole structure will always remain shaky. It can fall any day. New foundations are needed — everything new. You have to be completely reborn, otherwise it will be a modification. You can be painted from the outside, but there is no way to paint the inner. The inner will remain the same — the same old rotten thing.

A discontinuity is needed. You should not be allowed to continue. A gap. . . The old simply dies and the new comes out of it — out of the death. And there is a gap between the old and the new; otherwise the old can go on continuing. All modifications are really to save the old, and I am not a modifier. And the chaos will continue for you if you resist it. Then it takes a long time.

If you allow it to happen, it can happen in a single moment also. If you allow it to happen, the old disappears and a new being comes into being. That new will be divine because it will not come out of the past; it will not come out of time. It will be timeless—beyond time. It will not come out of you; you will not be a father and mother to it. It will come suddenly out of the blue.

That's why Buddha insists that it always come out of nothing. You are something; that is the misery. What you are in fact? Just the past. You go on accumulating the past; that's why you have become like ruins—very ancient ones. Just see the point and don't try to continue the old. Drop it!

Hence, around me there is going to be always chaos because I am continuously demolishing. I am destructive because that is the only way to be creative. I am like death because only then you can be born through me. It is right: there is chaos. There will always continue because new peoples will be coming. You will never find a settled establishment around me. New peoples will be coming and I will be demolishing them.

It can stop for you individually; if you allow me to destroy you completely, for you chaos will disappear. You will become a cosmos, a hidden harmony; a deep order. For you chaos will disappear, but around me it will continue because new ones will be coming. This has to be so; this has been always so.

It is not for the first time that you have asked me this. The same was asked to Buddha; the same was asked to Lao Tzu; the same will be asked again and again, because whenever there is a Master, that means he uses death as a method for resurrection. You must die; only then you can be reborn.

Chaos is beautiful because it is the womb, and your

so-called order is ugly because it protects only the dead. Death is beautiful; dead is not beautiful — remember the difference. Death is beautiful, I repeat, because death is a live force. Dead is not beautiful because dead is that place from where life has moved already. It is just a ruin. Don't be a dead one; don't carry the past. Drop it, and pass through death. You are afraid of death, but you are not afraid of dead.

Jesus called two fishermen to follow him, and the moment they were getting out of the town a man came running, and he said to the fishermen, "Where are you going? Your father has died. Come back." They asked Jesus, "Allow us few days so that we can go and do whatsoever is needed. Our father is dead and the last rituals have to be done." Jesus said, "Let the dead bury their dead. You don't bother. You follow me." What Jesus says? He says the whole town is dead; they will take care: "Let the dead bury their dead. You follow me."

If you live in the past you are a dead thing. You are not an alive force. And there is only one way to become alive, and that is to die to the past, die to the dead. And this is not going to happen once and forever. Once you know the secret, each moment you have to die to the past, so no dust gathers on you. Then death becomes a constant reorientation, a constant rebirth.

Always remember: die to the past! Whatsoever has passed, has passed. It is no more; it is nowhere. It only clings in the memory. It is only in your mind. Mind is the depository of all that is dead. That's why mind is the only block for life to flow. The dead bodies accumulate around the flow; they become the block.

All that I am doing here is in helping you to learn how to die because that's the first aspect of how to be reborn. Death is beautiful because life comes out of it fresh like dewdrops. So chaos is being used, and you will feel around me, and that will always be so, because somewhere or other somebody I am demolishing. In thousands of ways — known to you, unknown to you —

I am demolishing you. I am shaking you out of your death, shaking you out of your past, trying to make you more aware and more alive.

In the old ancient Hindu scriptures it is said that a Master is a death. They knew that a Master has to be death, because out of that death—revolution, mutation, transformation, transcendence. Death is an alchemy: it is the most subtle alchemy. Nature uses it. When somebody becomes very old and ancient, nature kills him.

You are afraid because you cling to the past. Otherwise you will be happy and you will welcome, and you will feel grateful to nature because always the old, the past, the dead, nature kills, and your life moves into a new body.

An old man becomes a new baby completely clean of the past. That's why nature helps you not to remember the past. Nature uses ways not to allow you to remember the past; otherwise you will be old the very moment you are born. Because the old man dies and is born as a new baby, so if he can remember the past he will be already old; the whole purpose will be lost.

Nature closes the past for you, so every birth seems to be a new birth. But you again start accumulating. When it is too much, nature will kill you again. One becomes capable to know his past lives only when one is dead to the past. Then nature opens the door. Then nature knows; now there is no need for nature to hide from you. You have attained to the constant newness, freshness of life. Now you know how to die: nature need not kill you.

Once you know that you are not the past, you are not the future but you are the very "presentness" of things, then whole nature opens its doors and mysteries. Your whole past—millions of lives lived in many, many ways—all reveal. Now it can be revealed because you will not be burdened by it. Now no past can burden you. And if you have come to know the alchemy of how to become continuously new, this will be your last life, because then there is no need to kill you and help you to be reborn. There is no need! You are doing it yourself every moment.

That is the meaning why a Buddha disappears and never comes back, why an enlightened person is never born again; that is the secret: because he knows now death, and he uses it continuously. Every moment, whatsoever is past, is passed and dead, and he is freed of it. Every moment he dies to the past and is born anew. It becomes a flow, a river-like flow of gaining fresh life every moment. Then there is no need for nature to gather seventy years nonsense, rubbish, rot, and then kill this ruin of a man, and help him to be born again, and to put him in the same circle, because he will gather again.

This is a vicious circle. Hindus have called it the *sansar*. *Sansar* means the wheel: the wheel goes on moving again and again on the same route. An enlightened person is one who has dropped out — out of the wheel. He says, "No more of it! Nature need not kill me because now I kill myself every moment."

And if you are fresh, nature need not use death for you, but then there is no need for birth also, because you are using birth continuously. Every moment you die to the past and are born to the present. That's why you feel a subtle freshness around a Buddha, as if he has taken a bath just now. You come near him and you feel a fragrance — a fragrance of freshness. You can never meet the same Buddha again. Every moment he is new.

Hindus are very wise because thousands of years of encountering Buddhas, *Jinas* — conquerors of life, enlightened, awakened people, they have realized many truths. One of the truths you will see all around. No Buddha is depicted as old, no Mahavira is depicted as old. No statue, no picture exists; Krishna, Ram, Buddha, Mahavira, nobody, is depicted as old.

Not that they never became old: they became old. Buddha became old when he was eighty years. He was as old as anybody will become when he is eighty, but he is not depicted as old. The reason is inner: because whenever you will come near him, you will find him young and fresh. So the oldness was just on the body, not on him. And I have to demolish you because your body may be young, but your inner being is very very old and ancient, a ruin, just like the Greek ruins of Persepolis and others.

Inside you, you have a ruin of being; it has to be demolished, and I have to be a furnace, a fire, a death to you. That's the only way I can help and bring a cosmos within you, an order. And I am not working to enforce any order upon you because that won't help. Any order enforced from without will be just a propping thing for the old ancient ruin: it will not help.

I believe in an inner order. That happens with your own awareness and rebirth. That comes from within and spreads outwards. Just like a flower, it opens, and the petals move outwards from the center to the periphery. Only that order is real and beautiful which opens within you and spreads all around you. If order is enforced from without, a discipline given to you—"Do this and don't do that"—and you are forced to be a prisoner, that won't help because it won't change you.

Nothing can change from the outside. There is only one revolution, and that is that which comes from the within. But before that revolution happens you must be destroyed utterly. Only on your grave the new will be born. That's why there is chaos around me: because I am a chaos! And I am using chaos as a method.

The second question:

*In doing* sadhana *on Aum, is it better to repeat it like a mantra or to try to hear it as an inner sound?*

The mantra Aum has to be done in three stages. First, you should repeat it very loudly. That means it should come from the body — first from the body because body is the main door. And let first the body be saturated with it.

So repeat it loudly. Move to a temple or in your room or somewhere where you can repeat it as loudly as you like. Use the whole body to repeat it, as if thousands of people are listening to you without microphone, and you have to be very loud so that the whole body trembles, shakes with it. And for few months, almost three months, you should not bother about anything else. The first stage is very important because it gives the foundation. Loudly, as if your every cell of the body is crying it, chanting it. . .

After three months, when you feel your body is completely saturated, deep down it has entered into the body cells. And when you say it loudly, it is not only the mouth: from head to toe, the whole body is repeating it. It comes! If for three months you repeat it continuously at least one hour per day, within three months you will feel that it is not the mouth, it is the whole body. It happens — it has happened many times!

If you do it really honestly, authentically, and are not deceiving yourself, it is not lukewarm but a hundred-degree phenomenon, then even others can listen. They can put their ears to your feet, and when you say loudly they will listen it from your bones coming because the whole body can absorb sound and the whole body can create sound. There is no problem about it. Your mouth is just a part of the body — a specialized part, that's all. If you try, your whole body can repeat it.

It happened: one Hindu sannyasin, Swami Ram, did it for many years, loudly chanting "Ram". Once he was staying in a Himalayan village with a friend. The friend was a very well-known Sikh writer, Sardar Purnasingh.

In the middle of the night Purnasingh suddenly heard a chanting of "Ram, Ram, Ram". There was nobody else — only Ram, Swami Ram, and himself. They both were sleeping on their cots, and the village was far away — almost two, three miles away. There was nobody.

So Purnasingh got up, went around the cottage; there is nobody. And the more he went further from Ram, the sound was lesser and lesser. When he came back, the sound was again more. Then he came nearer Ram who was fast asleep. The moment he came nearer, the sound became even more loud. Then he put his ear to Ram's body. The whole body was vibrating with the sound of "Ram".

It happens. Your whole body can become saturated. This is the first step — three months, six months — but you must feel saturated. And the saturation is felt just like when you are hungry you take food — you feel when the stomach is satisfied. The body must be satisfied first, and if you continue, it may happen in three months or six months. Three months is the average limit; to few people it happens even before; to few it takes a little time more.

If it saturates the whole body, sex will disappear completely. The whole body is so soothed, it becomes so calm with the sound vibrating, that there is no need to throw the energy out, there is no need to release, and you will feel very, very powerful. But don't use this power — because you can use, and all use will be misuse — because this is just a first step.

Energy has to be gathered so that you can take the second step. If you use it. . . You can use — because the power will be so much you can do many things — you can simply say something and it will come true. At this stage it has been prohibited that you should not be active, and you should not say anything. You should not say somebody in anger that "Go and die," because this can happen. Your sound becomes so powerful when it is saturated with your whole body energy, so it is said at this stage no negative thing should be said — even unknowingly. No negative thing should be said!

You may be surprised, but it is good I should tell you: we were making a roof at the back of this house; it fell down. It fell down because of many of you. You are doing tremendous effort in meditation, and there were at least twenty persons who were thinking that it will fall. They helped: they helped it to fall. At least twenty persons were thinking continuously. . . When they were there, they will look at it, they will think it will fall, because the shape was such that it was unlikely to their minds that it is going to remain.

It fell! And when it fell, they thought, "Of course! we were right." This is the vicious circle. You are the cause and you think you were right. And you are all doing much effort in meditation. Whatsoever you think, can happen. Never think a negative thought when you are meditating. It is possible because you gain some power. But I am not concerned with the roof that it fell. Because of this falling many of you have lost a certain quantity of power; that is more a concern to me because nothing happens without your power used in it.

Those who were saying that it will fall. . .the roof fell. And they can watch themselves. For few days they remained very impotent, sad, depressed. They lost their power. They may be thinking they are sad because the roof has fallen — no! They were sad because they have lost a certain quantity of power, and life is an energy phenomenon.

When you don't meditate, there is not much problem. You can say whatsoever you like because you are impotent. But when you meditate, you should be watchful of every single word that you say because your every single word can create something around.

First step is to saturate the whole body, so the whole body becomes a chanting force. When you feel satisfied, then take the second step. And never use this power because this power has to be accumulated and to be used for the second step.

The second step is to close your mouth and repeat and chant the word Aum mentally — first bodily, second mentally. Now the body should not be used at all. The throat, the tongue, the lips, everything, closed, the whole body locked and chanting only in the mind — but as loudly as possible: the same loudness as you were using with the body. Now let the mind saturate with it. Three months again, let the mind saturate with it.

The same time will taken by the mind as it has been taken by the body. If you can attain the saturation within one month with the body, you will attain with one month in the mind also. If you attain in seven months with the body, seven months will be taken by the mind, because body and mind are not exactly two. They are rather body-mind — psychosomatic phenomenon. One part is body, another part is mind: body is visible mind, mind is invisible body.

So let the other part, the subtle part of your personality, be saturated; repeat inside loudly. When the mind is filled, even more power is released within you. With the first, sex will disappear; with the second, love will disappear — the love that you know, not the love that a Buddha knows, but your love will disappear.

Because sex is the bodily part of love and love is the mental part of sex. When love disappears, then there is even more danger. You can be very, very fatal to others. If you say something, it will immediately happen. That's why, for the second state, total silence is proposed. When you are in the second stage, be completely silent.

And there will be a tendency to use the power, because you will be very curious about it, childish. And you will have so much energy that you would like to see what can happen. But don't use it and don't be juvenile, because the third step has to be still taken and energy is needed. That's why sex disappeared — because energy has to be accumulated: love disappeared—because subtle energy has to be accumulated.

And the third step is when the mind feels saturated. And you will come to know it when this happens; there is no need to ask how one will feel it. It is just like eating: you feel, "Now, enough!" The mind will feel when it is enough. Then you start the third step. The third is: neither body has to be used nor mind has to be used. As you lock the body, now you lock the mind.

And it is easy. When you have been doing the chanting for three, four months, it is very easy: you simply lock the body, you simply lock the mind. Just listen, and you will hear a sound coming to you from your own heart of hearts. The Aum will be there as if somebody else is chanting; you are just the listener. This is the third step, and this third step will change your total being. All the barriers will drop and all the obstacles will disappear. So it can take almost nine months, average, if you put your total energy in it.

*In doing sadhana on Aum is it better to repeat it like a mantra or to try to hear it as an inner sound?*

Right now you cannot hear it as an inner sound. The inner sound is there, but it is so silent, so subtle, and you don't have that ear to listen to it. The ear has to be developed. The body saturated, the mind saturated, only then you will have that ear—the third ear, so to say—that you can listen to the sound which is there always.

It is a cosmic sound; it is in and out. Put your ear to the tree and it is there; put your ear to the rock and it is there. But first your body-mind should be transcended, and you should gain more and more energy. The subtle will require tremendous energy to be heard.

With the first sex disappears, with the second step love disappears and with the third step everything that you have known disappears, as if you are no more—

dead, gone, dissolved. It is a death phenomenon, and if you don't escape and become scared, because there will be every tendency in you to escape, because this looks like an abyss, and you are falling into it and the abyss is bottomless. . . There seems to be no end to it. You become like a feather falling into a bottomless abyss — falling and falling and falling — and there seems to be no end to it.

You will get scared. You would like to run away from it. If you run away from it, the whole effort has been a wastage. And the running will be that you will start chanting the mantra Aum: that will be the first thing to do if you start running, because if you chant you are back into the mind. If you chant loudly you are back into the body.

So when one starts listening one should not chant, because that chanting will be an escape. A mantra has to be chanted and then dropped. A mantra is complete only when you can drop it. If you go on chanting it, you will cling to it like a shelter, and whenever you will be afraid, you will come again and chant it.

That's why I say chant it so deeply that the body is saturated; there is no need to chant in the body again. The mind is saturated, there is no need to chant it; overflowing, there is no space to put more chanting into it. So you cannot escape. Only then the hearing of the soundless sound becomes possible.

Another friend has asked that:

*Before, you used to talk about the mantra Hoo. Then why you are emphasizing now the mantra Aum?*

I am not emphasizing. I am simply explaining to you Patanjali. My emphasis remains for Hoo. And whatsoever I am saying about Aum, the same is applicable to Hoo. But my emphasis remains with Hoo.

As I told you, Patanjali existed five thousand years before. People were simple — very simple, innocent.

They could trust easily; they had not much of the mind. They were not head oriented: they were heart oriented. Aum is a mild sound—soothing, non-violent, non-aggressive. If you chant Aum, it goes from the throat to the heart, never below it. Those were heart people— Aum was enough for them: a mild dose, a homeopathic dose, was enough for them.

For you, it won't help much. For you, Hoo will be more helpful. Hoo is a Sufi mantra. Just like Aum is a Hindu mantra, Hoo is a Mohammedan, Sufi mantra. Hoo was developed by Sufis for a country and race very aggressive, violent—not simple people, not innocent— cunning and clever, fighters. For them Hoo was invented.

Hoo is the last part of Allah. If you repeat "Allah-Allah-Allah-Allah" continuously, by and by, it takes the shape of "Allahoo-Allahoo-Allahoo". Then, by and by, the first part is to be dropped. It becomes "Lahoo-Lahoo-Lahoo". Then even "Lah" is to be dropped. It becomes "Hoo-Hoo-Hoo". It is very forceful, and it hits your sex center directly. It doesn't hit your heart: it hits your sex center.

For you Hoo will be helpful because now your heart is almost non-functioning. Love has disappeared; only sex has remained. Your sex center is functioning, not your love center, so Aum will not be of much help. Hoo will be a deeper help because your energy is not now near the heart. Your energy is near the sex center, and the sex center has to be hit directly so the energy rises upwards.

After a period of doing Hoo, you may feel that now you don't need that much of a dose. Then you can turn over to Aum. When you start feeling that now you exist near the heart, not near the sex center, only then can you use Aum—not before it. But there is no need: Hoo can do the whole way.

But if you feel like, you can change. If you feel that now there is no need, you don't feel like sexual—sex is not a worry to you, you don't think about it; it is not a cerebral imagination, you are not fascinated by it; a beautiful woman passes and you simply take a note that "Yes, a woman has passed," but nothing arises within you; your sex center is not hit, no energy moves in you —then you can start Aum.

But no need: you can continue with Hoo. Hoo is a stronger dose. When you do Hoo, you can immediately feel it goes to the stomach—to the center of *hara*, and then to the sex center. It forces the sex energy immediately upwards. It stirs the sex center.

And you are more head oriented. This always happens: people, countries, civilizations which are head oriented become sexual—more sexual than heart oriented people. Heart oriented people are loving. Sex comes as a shadow of love; it is not important in itself. Heart oriented people don't think much because, really, if you watch twenty-four hours, twenty-three hours you are thinking about sex.

Heart oriented people don't think about sex at all. When it happens, it happens. It is just like a body need. And it follows as a shadow to love: it never happens directly. They live in the middle—the heart is the middle between head and sex centers—you live in the head and in the sex. You move from these two extremes; you are never in the middle. When the sex is fulfilled, you move to the heart. When the sex desire arises, you move to the sex but you never stay in the middle. The pendulum moves right and left—never stops in the middle.

Patanjali developed this method of chanting Aum for very simple people—innocent villagers living with nature. For you. . . You can try it; if it helps, it is good. But my understanding about you is this, that it will not help more than one percent of you. Ninety-nine percent will be helped by the mantra Hoo. It is nearer you.

And, remember, when the mantra Hoo succeeds, when you reach to the listening point, you will listen

*Aumkar*, not Hoo. You will listen Aum! The final phenomenon will be the same. It is just on the path. . .you
are difficult people. Stronger doses are needed, that's
all. But on the final stay, you will experience the same
phenomenon.

My emphasis remains for Hoo because my emphasis
depends not on Hindus or Mohammedans; my emphasis
depends on you, what is your need. I am neither a
Hindu nor a Mohammedan. I am nobody, so I am free. I
can use anything from anywhere. A Hindu will feel
guilty using Allah; a Mohammedan will feel guilty using
Aum: but I am not fussy about such things. If Allah
helps, it is beautiful; if *Aumkar* helps, it is beautiful. I
bring every method to you according to your need.

To me, all religions lead to the same; the goal is one.
And all religions are like paths leading to the same
summit. On the top, everything becomes one. Now it
depends on you — where you are — and which path will
be nearer. Aum will be very far from you; Hoo is very
nearer. It is your need. My emphasis depends on your
need. My emphasis is not theoretical; it is not sectarian.
My emphasis is absolutely personal. I look at you and
decide.

The fourth question:

*You said that needs are to do with the body and
desires are to do with the mind. Which of these
two brought us to you?*

Before I answer this, one thing more has to be understood; then it will be possible for you to understand the
answer to this question. You are not only body and
mind: you are something else also — the soul, the self —
the *atman*. Body has needs, the *atman* also has needs;
just between the two is the mind which has desires.

Body has needs—hunger to be satisfied, thirst. A shelter is needed, food is needed, water is needed. Body has needs; the mind has desires. Nothing is needed, but mind creates false needs.

A desire is a false need. If you don't attend to it, you feel frustrated, a failure. If you attend to it, nothing is attained because in the first place, it was never a need: it never existed as a need.

You can fulfill a need; you cannot fulfill a desire. Desire is a dream—a dream cannot be fulfilled; it has no roots, neither in the earth, nor in the sky. It has no roots! Mind is a dreaming phenomenon. You ask for fame, name, prestige: even if you attain you will not attain anything because fame will not satisfy any need. It is not a need. You may become famous. If the whole earth knows about you, what—what then? What will happen to you? What can you do with it? It is neither food nor drink. When the whole world knows you, you feel frustrated. What to do with it? It is useless.

Soul has needs again. Just as body has a need for food, soul has a need for food. Of course, the food is God then. You must remember Jesus saying to his disciples many times, "Eat me. I am your food. And let me be your drink." What he means?—a different need. Unless it is satisfied, unless you can eat God, unless you become God by eating him, absorbing him—he flows in your soul like blood, He becomes your consciousness—you will remain unsatisfied.

The soul has needs: religion fulfills those needs. The body has needs: science fulfills those needs. Mind has desires or tries to fulfill, but cannot fulfill. It is just a boundary land where body and soul meet. When body and soul are separate, mind simply disappears. It has no existence of its own.

Now take this question:

*You said that needs are to do with the body and desires are to do with the mind. Which of these two brought us to you?*

There are three types of persons here around me: one who have come because of their body needs. They are frustrated with sex, frustrated with love, miserable in the body. They have come, they can be helped; their problem is honest, and once their body needs disappear, their soul needs will arise.

Then there is a second group who has come because of the soul needs. They can be helped because they have real needs. They have come not for their sex problems, love problems or body diseases, illnesses. They have not come for that. They have come to seek the truth; they have come to enter the mystery of life; they have come to know what this existence is.

And then there is a third group, and the third is greater of these both two. Those people have come because of their mind desires. They cannot be helped. They will hang around me for some time and then disappear. Or, if they hang around me a longer period, then I may reduce them either to body needs or to soul needs, but their mind needs cannot be fulfilled because they are not needs in the first place.

There are few persons who are here for egoistic reasons. Sannyas is an ego trip for them. They become special, extraordinary. They have failed in life: they couldn't attain to political power, they couldn't reach to wordly fame, they couldn't achieve wealth, material things. They feel nobodies. Now I give them sannyas, and without anything on their part, they become somebody important, special. Just by changing to orange, they think now they are not ordinary people—they are the chosen few, different from everybody else. They will go in the world and condemn everybody, that "You are just worldly creatures! Absolutely wrong you are. We are the saved ones, the chosen few."

These are mind desires. Remember not to be here for any mind desire. Otherwise you are simply wasting your time: they cannot be fulfilled. I am here to bring you out of your dreams; I am not here to fulfill your dreams. These people will bring all types of politics here because they are on the ego trip. They will bring all sorts of conflicts; they will create cliques. They will create a miniature world here, and they will create a hierarchy, that, "I am higher than you, holier than you." They will play the game of one-upmanship.

But they are fools. They should not be here in the first place. They have chosen a wrong place for their ego trips because I am here to kill their egos completely, to shatter them. That's why you feel so much chaos around me. Remember, you can be in a right place for wrong reasons. Then you miss, because the question is not the place; the question is why you are here. If you are for your body needs, something can be done, and when your body needs are settled, your soul needs will arise.

If you are here for mind needs, drop those needs. They are not needs; they are dreams. Drop them as completely as possible. And don't ask how to drop them because nothing is to be done for them to drop. Just the very understanding that they are mind desires, is enough: they drop automatically.

The fifth question:

*Is it possible to find a synthesis between yoga and tantra? Does one lead to another?*

No, it is impossible. It is as impossible as if you try to find a synthesis between man and woman. Then what will be the synthesis? — third sex, an impotent person, will be the synthesis and that will neither be man nor woman. Rootless, that man will nowhere be. . .

Tantra is absolutely opposite, diametrically opposite than yoga. You cannot make any synthesis. And never try such things because you will be more and more confused. One is enough to confuse you; two will be too much. And they lead in different directions. They reach to the same summit; they reach to the same peak. Synthesis is there at the top, at the climax, but at the foothill, where the journey starts, they are absolutely different. One goes to the east, another goes to the west. They say goodbye to each other; they have their backs to each other. They are like man and woman — different psychologies, beautiful in their difference.

If you make a synthesis, it becomes ugly. A woman has to be a woman — so much of a woman that she becomes a polarity to man. In their polarities they are beautiful because in their polarities they are attracted to each other. In their polarities they are complementary, but you cannot synthesize. Synthesis will be just poor, synthesis will be just powerless. There will be no tension in it.

At the peak they meet, and that meeting is orgasm. Where man and woman meet, when their bodies dissolve, when they are not two things, when yin and yang are one, it becomes one circle of energy. For a moment, at the summit of bio-energy, they meet and then they fall again.

The same is with tantra and yoga. Tantra is feminine, yoga is male. Tantra is surrender, yoga is will. Tantra is effortlessness, yoga is effort — tremendous effort. Tantra is passive, yoga is active. Tantra is like the earth, yoga is like the sky. They meet, but there is no synthesis. They meet at the top, but at the foothill where the journey starts, where you all are standing, you have to choose the path.

Paths cannot be synthesized. And people who try that, they confuse humanity. They confuse very deeply and they are not a help; they are very harmful. Paths cannot be synthesized — only the end. Path has to be separate from another path — perfectly separate, different in its very tone, being. When you follow tantra, you move through sex. That is tantra's path; you allow nature a total surrender. It is a let-go, you don't fight, it is not a path of a warrior. You don't struggle; you surrender wherever nature leads. Nature leads into sex, you surrender to sex. You completely move into it with no guilt, with no concept of sin.

Tantra has no concept of sin, no guilt. Move into sex. Just remain alert, watching what is happening. Be alert, mindful what is going on. But don't try to control, don't try to contain yourself; allow the flow. Move into the woman; let the woman move into you. Let them become a circle and you remain a watcher. Through this watching and let-go, tantra achieves a transcendence. Sex disappears. This is one way to go beyond nature because going beyond sex is going beyond nature.

Whole nature is sexual. Flowers are there because they are sexual. All beauty exists because of some sexual phenomenon. A continuous game is on. Trees are attracting others, birds are calling others. Everywhere a sexual game is on. Nature is sex, and to achieve to the supersex is to go beyond sex. But tantra says use sex as a step. Don't fight with it: go beyond it, using it. Move through it, pass through it, and attain to the transcendence through experience. A watchful experience becomes transcendence.

Yoga says don't waste energy: bypass sex completely. No need to go into it: you can simply bypass. Conserve energy, and don't be befooled by nature. Fight nature, become a willpower; become a controlled being not floating anywhere. The whole yoga methods are how to make you capable so that there is no need to let go into the nature, no need to allow nature to have its own way. You become a master and you move on your own against nature, fighting nature. It is a way of the warrior —the impeccable warrior who continuously fights, and through fighting transcends.

These are totally different. Both lead to the same goal: choose one; don't try to synthesize. How can you synthesize? If you go through sex, yoga is dropped.

How can you synthesize? If you leave sex, tantra is dropped. How can you synthesize? But remember, both lead to the same goal: transcendence is the goal. It depends on you — on your type. Are you a warrior type, a man who fights continuously? Then yoga is your path. If you are not a warrior type, if you are passive — in a subtle way feminine, you would not like to fight with anybody, really non-violent — then tantra is the path, and because both lead to the same goal, there is no need to synthesize.

Synthesizers, to me, are always almost wrong. All Gandhis are wrong; whosoever synthesizes is wrong, because it is synthesizing allopathy with ayurvedic; it is synthesizing homeopathy with allopathic; it is synthesizing with Hindu and Mohammedan; it is synthesizing Buddha and Patanjali. No need to synthesize! Each path in itself is perfect! Each path in itself is so perfect, it doesn't need anything to be added to it; and any addition can be dangerous because a part may be functioning in a particular machine. . .may become a barrier into another.

You can take a part from an Impala car. It was functioning well into it, and you can put it into a Ford and it may create problems. A part functions in a pattern. A part depends on the pattern, on the whole. You cannot use simply a part anywhere. And what these synthesizers do? They take one part from one system, another part from another system; they make a hodge-podge, and if you follow these fellows you will become a hodge-podge. No need to synthesize. Just try to find out your type, feel your type, and there is no hurry; watch and feel your type.

Can you surrender? — surrender to nature? — then surrender. If you feel it is impossible, "I cannot surrender", then don't be depressed because there is another path which needs no surrender in this way, which gives you all opening to fight. And both lead to the same at the peak, when you have reached the Gourishankar. By and by, as you reach nearer and nearer to the peak, you see others are also reaching who were traveling on different paths.

Ramakrishna tried one of the greatest experiments in the whole history of humanity. When he became enlightened, after his enlightenment, he tried many paths. Nobody has done that ever because there is no need. You have attained to the peak; why be worried whether other paths lead to it or not? But Ramakrishna did a great service to humanity. He came back down to the foothill again and tried another path—whether it also leads to the top or not. He tried many, and each time he reached to the same point.

This is his simile—that at the foothill, paths are different. They move in different directions, even look opposite, contradictory. But at the top they meet; synthesis is at the top. At the beginning, diversions, multiplicity; in the end, unity, oneness.

Don't bother about synthesis. You simply choose your path and stick to it. And don't be allured by others who will be calling to you to come to their path because it leads. Hindus have reached, Mohammedans have reached, Jews have reached, Christians have reached, and the ultimate truth has no conditioning that if you are a Hindu only then you will reach.

The only thing to be worried about is to feel your type and choose. I am not against anything; I am for everything. Whatsoever you choose, I can help you that way. But no synthesis! Don't try for synthesis.

The sixth question:

*Often when you are talking to us, waves of energy come to us opening our hearts and bringing tears of gratitude. You have said that*

*you fill us whenever we are open, but often this
phenomenon happens to many people at the
same time, like shaktipat. Why do you not give
us this wonderful experience more often?*

It is up to you. It is not that I am giving any experience
to you. It is up to you; you can take it. It is not a giving
because I am giving all the time. It is for you to be open
and take it. And this is right, that it happens many times
to many people together. Then the logical mind says I
must be doing something; otherwise, why to so many
people it is happening together?

No, I am not doing. But when one opens, the opening
of one is infectious. Others immediately start opening.
It is just like one starts coughing and others start coughing; it is infectious. One opens: you suddenly feel something is happening around; you also become open.

I am available continuously. Whenever you open,
you can share me. Whenever you are closed, you cannot share. And it is not for me; it is up to you to do
something. Of course it happens together, because one
opens another, and then it goes on and on. It can become a flood-like phenomenon.

In Indonesia there is a particular method known as
*latihan.* They use the word *opening:* one who is open
can open others. The Master, one of the very, very
significant men upon this earth right now, the Master of
*latihan,* is a man called Bapak Subud. He has opened
few people, and then he tells those people to go around
the earth and open others.

And what they do? They do a very simple method.
You will be able to understand it because you are doing
many methods on the similar lines. One who is opened
by Bapak Subud moves with a newcomer—one who is
to be opened—the disciple. They stand in a closed
room. The one who is already open, he raises his hands
towards the sky. He opens himself, and the other simply

stands there. Within a few minutes the other starts trembling. Something is happening, and when he is opened, opened to the infinite sky, to the infinite energy from the beyond, now he is allowed to open others.

And nobody knows what they do; even the doer never knows what he is doing. He simply stands there and the other is just standing nearby—the neophyte. And they don't know. . .they ask Bapak Subud, "What is this?" They do it—it happens—but Bapak Subud never gives any explanation. He is not that type of man. He says, "You simply do. Don't bother why it happens. It happens!"

The same happens here. One opens. Suddenly, the energy moves around him; he creates a milieu. You are near him; suddenly you feel a surge coming up, tears start flowing, your heart is full. You open; you help another. . . It becomes a chain reaction. The whole world can be opened; and once you are open, you know the knack of it. It is not a method; you simply know the knack of it. Then you simply put in a certain situation your mind, in a certain way your being: this is what I call prayer.

To me, prayer is not a verbal communication to the divine. Because how can you communicate with language with the divine? The divine has no language and whatsoever you say will not be understood. You can be understood not by language, but by your being. Being is the only language.

Try a small prayer method. In the night, when you are going to the bed, just kneel down near the bed. Put the light off, raise your both hands, close your eyes, and just feel as if you are under a waterfall—an energy waterfall from the sky. In the beginning, it is an imagination. In the beginning it has to be an imagination. Within two, three days you start feeling that it is a real phenomenon—you are under a waterfall—your body starts shaking, as if a leaf in a strong wind. And the fall is so strong and tremendous you cannot contain it; it fills you pore to pore, from toe to head. You have become just an empty vessel and it fills you.

When you feel trembling coming to you, cooperate with it. Help the trembling to grow more, because the more you tremble, the more is the possibility for the infinite energy to descend in you, because your own inner energy becomes dynamic. When you are dynamic, you can meet the dynamic force; when you are static, you cannot meet the dynamic force.

When you tremble, energy is created within you. Energy attracts more energy. Become a vessel — empty, filled, overflowing. When you feel now it is too much, unbearable, the fall is too much and you cannot bear it any more, bow down to the earth, kiss the earth and remain silent there as if you are pouring the energy into the earth.

Take from the sky; give back to the earth. You become just a medium in between. Bow down completely; become empty again. When you feel now you are empty, you will feel so silent, so calm, so collected! Then raise your hands again. Feel the energy. Go down, kiss the earth: give the energy back to the earth.

Energy is sky, energy is earth. There are two types of energy: sky is always called the male because it gives, and earth is always called the female because it takes, it is like a womb. So take from the sky and give to the earth. And this has to be done seven times — not less — because each time the energy will penetrate one chakra of your body, and there are seven chakras.

Each time the energy will go deeper in you; it will stir a deeper core within you. Seven times is a must. Less you should not do because if you do less you will not be able to sleep. Energy will be there inside and you will feel restless. Do it seven times. More you can do, more there is no harm, but less not! — do it seven times or more.

And when you feel completely empty, go to sleep. Your whole night will become a happening. In sleep, you will become more and more silent. Dreams will stop. In the morning, you will feel a completely new being arising, resurrected. You are no more the old. The past is dropped; you are fresh and young.

Every night do it. Within three months many things will become possible. You will be open, and then you can open others. After doing three months this opening phenomenon, you can simply stand by the side of somebody and open yourself, and immediately you will feel that the other is shaking, trembling. Even if he doesn't know, even without his knowing you can open somebody. But don't do that because the other will be simply scared. He will think that something weird is happening.

Once opened, you can open others. It is an affection, and a beautiful infection: an infection of perfect health, not of any disease — an infection of wholeness, infection of holiness, infection of the sacred.

# Cultivating Right Attitudes

*The mind becomes tranquil by cultivating attitudes of friendliness towards the happy, compassion towards the miserable, joy towards the virtuous and indifference towards the evil.*

*The mind also becomes tranquil by alternately expelling and retaining the breath.*

*When meditation produces extraordinary sense perceptions, the mind gains confidence and this helps perseverance.*

*Also, meditate on the inner light which is serene and beyond all sorrow.*

*Also meditate on one who has attained desirelessness.*

*The mind becomes tranquil by cultivating attitudes of friendliness towards the happy, compassion towards the miserable, joy towards the virtuous and indifference towards the evil.*

MANY THINGS HAVE TO be understood before you can understand this sutra. First, the natural attitudes: whenever you see somebody happy, you feel jealous—not happy, never happy. You feel miserable. That's the natural attitude, the attitude that you have already got.

And Patanjali says the mind becomes tranquil by cultivating attitudes of friendliness towards the happy —
very difficult. To be friendly with someone who is
happy is one of the most difficult things in life.

Ordinarily, you think it is very easy. It is not! Just
the opposite is the case. You feel jealous, you feel miserable. You may show happiness, but that's just a facade,
a show, a mask. And how you can be happy? And how
you can be tranquil, silent, if you have such an attitude?

Because the whole life is celebrating, millions of hap-
pinesses happening all over the universe, but if you have
an attitude of jealousy, you will be miserable, you will
be in a constant hell. And you will be in a hell precisely
because all over there is heaven. You will create a hell
for you — a private hell — because whole existence is
celebrating.

If somebody is happy, what comes first to your
mind? — as if that happiness has been taken from you, as
if he has won and you are defeated, as if he has cheated
you. . . Happiness is not a competition, so don't be worried. If somebody is happy, it does not mean that you
cannot be happy, that he has taken happiness — now
how you can be happy. Happiness is not somewhere
existing, which can be exhausted by happy people.

Why you feel jealous? If somebody is rich, maybe it
is difficult for you to be rich because riches exist in a
quantity. If somebody is powerful in a material way, it
may be difficult for you to be powerful because power is
a competition. But happiness is not a competition. Happiness exists in infinite quantity. Nobody has ever been
able to exhaust it; there is no competition at all. If somebody is happy, why you feel jealous? And with jealousy
enters hell in you.

Says Patanjali, when somebody is happy, feel happy,
feel friendly. Then you also open a door towards happiness. In a subtle way, if you can feel friendly with someone who is happy, you immediately start sharing his
happiness; it has become yours also — immediately! And

happiness is not some*thing*; it is not material. It is not something that somebody can cling to. You can share it. When a flower blooms, you can share it; when a bird sings, you can share it; when somebody is happy, you can share it. And the beauty is that it does not depend on his sharing. It depends on your partaking.

If it depended on his sharing, whether he shares or not, then it was totally a different thing. He may not like to share. But this is not a question at all; it does not depend on his sharing. When the sun rises in the morning you can be happy, and the sun cannot do anything about it. It cannot prevent you being happy. Somebody is happy: you can be friendly. It is totally your own attitude, and he cannot prevent you by sharing. Immediately you open a door, and his happiness flows towards you also.

This is the secret of creating a heaven all around you, and only within heaven can you be tranquil. How can you be tranquil in hell-fire? And nobody is creating it: you create it. So the basic thing to be understood is that whenever there is misery, hell, you are the cause of it. Never throw the responsibility on anybody else because that throwing of responsibility is escaping from the basic truth.

If you are miserable, only you—absolutely only you—are responsible. Look within and find the cause of it. And nobody wants to be miserable. If you can find the cause within you, you can throw it out. Nobody is standing in your way to prevent you. There is not a single obstacle to be happy.

But by being friendly towards happy people, you become attuned to happiness. They are flowering; you become friendly. They may not be friendly; that is none of your concern. They may not even know you—that doesn't matter. But wherever there is a blooming, wherever there is bliss, wherever somebody is flowering, wherever somebody is dancing and is happy and is smiling, wherever there is celebration, you become friendly, you partake of it. It starts flowing within you, and nobody can prevent it. And when there is happiness all around you, you feel tranquil.

*The mind becomes tranquil by cultivating attitudes of friendliness towards the happy. . .*

With the happy, you feel jealous—in a subtle competition. With happy people, you feel yourself inferior. You always choose people around you who are unhappy. You become friendly with unhappy people because with unhappy people you feel superior. You always seek somebody who is below you. You are always afraid of the higher; you always seek the lower, and the more you seek the lower, the lower you fall. Then even more lower people are needed.

Seek the company of those who are higher than you —higher in wisdom, higher in happiness, higher in tranquility, calmness, quiet, collectedness: always seek the company of the higher because that is the way how you become higher, how you transcend the valleys and reach to the peaks. That becomes a ladder. Always seek the company of the higher, the beautiful, the happy— you will become more beautiful, you will become more happy.

And once the secret is known, once you know how one becomes more happy, how with others' happiness you create a situation for yourself also to be happy, then there is no barrier; then you can go as far as you like. You can become a god where no unhappiness exists.

Who is a god? A god is one who has learned the secret to be happy with the whole universe, with every flower and with every river and with every rock and every star, who has become one with this continuous eternal celebration, who celebrates, who doesn't bother whose celebration is this. Wherever there is a celebration, he participates. This art of participating in happiness is one of the foundations if you want to be happy. It has to be followed.

Just the opposite you have been doing: if somebody is happy, immediately you are shocked. How is it possible? How come you are not happy and he has become happy? There is injustice. This whole world is cheating you and there is no God. If God is, how come you are not happy and others are becoming happy? And these people who are happy, they are the exploiters, they are tricky, cunning. They live on your blood. They are sucking others' happiness.

Nobody is sucking anybody's happiness. Happiness is such a phenomenon, there is no need to suck it. It is an inner flowering; it doesn't come from the outside. Just by being happy with happy people you create the situation in which your own inner flower starts blooming:

> *The mind becomes tranquil by cultivating*
> *attitudes of friendliness. . .*

You create the attitude of enmity. You can feel friendly with a sad person, and you think it is very virtuous. You can feel friendly with someone who is depressed, in misery, and you think it is something religious, something moral you are doing, but what are you doing, you don't know.

Whenever you feel friendly with someone who is sad, depressed, unhappy, miserable, you create misery for you. It looks very irreligious, Patanjali's attitude. It is not, because when you will understand his whole standpoint you will see what he means. He is very scientific. He is not a sentimental person, and sentimentality won't help you.

One has to be very very clear:

> *. . .compassion towards the miserable. . .*

Not friendliness—compassion. Compassion is a different quality; friendliness is different. Friendliness means you are creating a situation in which you would like to be the same as the other person is, you would like to be

the same as your friend. Compassion means that someone has fallen from his state. You would like to help
him, but you would not like to be like him. You would
like to give him a hand; you would like to bring him up,
cheer him up. You would like to help him in every way,
but you would not like to be like him because that is
not a help.

Somebody is crying and weeping, and you sit by the
side and you start crying and weeping: are you helping
him? In what way? Somebody is miserable and you
become miserable; are you helping him? You may be
doubling his misery. He was alone miserable; now there
are two persons miserable. But in showing sympathy to
the miserable you are again playing a trick. Deep down,
when you show sympathy to the miserable — and remember, sympathy is not compassion; sympathy is
friendliness. When you show sympathy and friendliness
to a depressed, sad, miserable person, deep down you
are feeling happy. Always there is an undercurrent of
happiness. It has to be so because it is a simple arith-
metic: when somebody is happy, you feel miserable,
then how it is possible when somebody is miserable you
can feel unhappy? Somebody is happy you feel miserable; then somebody is unhappy, deep down you feel
very happy.

But you don't show it. Or, if you are observed acute-
ly even you show it — even in your sympathy there is a
subtle current of happiness. You feel good; you feel
cheered up really, that it is not you who is unhappy,
and you are in a position to show sympathy — and you
are higher, suprior.

People always feel good when they can show sympathy to others; they are always cheered. Deep down they
feel that they are not so miserable, thank God! When
somebody dies, immediately an undercurrent in you
comes that you are still alive, thank God. And you can
show sympathy and it costs nothing. Showing sympathy costs nothing, but compassion is a different thing.

Compassion means you would like to help the other person; you would like to do whatsoever can be done; you would like to help him to come out of his misery. You are not happy about it, but you are not miserable also.

And just between the two exists compassion: Buddha is in compassion. He will not feel miserable with you because that is not going to help anybody, and he will not feel happy because there is no point in feeling happy. How can you feel happy when somebody is miserable? But he cannot feel unhappy also because that is not going to help. He will feel compassion. Compassion exists just in between these two. Compassion means he would like to help you to come out of it. He is for you, compassion means, but against your misery; he loves you, but not your misery. He would like to bring you up, but not your misery with you.

When you are sympathetic you start loving the misery, not the man who is miserable. And if suddenly the man is cheered up and says, "Don't bother," you will feel shocked, because he never gave you a chance to be sympathetic and show him that how higher, superior and happy a being you are.

Don't be miserable with somebody who is miserable. Help him to come out of it. Never make misery an object of love; don't give any affection to misery, because if you give affection and you make it an object of love, you are opening a door for it. Sooner or later you will become miserable. Remain aloof. Compassion means remain aloof! Extend your hand, remain aloof, help—don't feel miserable, don't feel happy, because both are the same. When you feel miserable on the surface with somebody's misery, deep down runs the current of being happy. Both have to be dropped. Compassion will bring you tranquility of the mind.

Many people come to me; they are social reformers, revolutionaries, politicians, utopians, and they say, "How you can teach people meditation and silence when there is so much misery in the world?" They tell me, "This is selfish." They would like me to teach people to be miserable with others who are miserable. They don't know what they are saying but they feel very good — doing social work, social service, they feel very good. And if suddenly the world becomes a heaven, and God says, "Now everything will be okay," you will find the social reformers and revolutionaries in absolute misery, because they will have nothing to do.

Khalil Gibran has written a small parable. In a city, in a big city, there was a dog who was a preacher and a missionary, and he preached to other dogs that "Stop barking. We waste almost ninety-nine percent of our energy in barking unnecessarily. That's why we have not been evolving. Stop barking unnecessarily."

But it is difficult for dogs to stop barking. That is an in-built process. Really they feel happy only when they bark. It is a catharsis. They feel silent when they have barked. So, they listened to the leader — the revolutionary, the utopian, who was thinking of kingdom of gods, kingdom of dogs, somewhere in the coming future, where every dog is reformed and has become religious — no barking, no fighting, everything is silent. . .a pacifist, must have been — that missionary.

But dogs are dogs. They will listen to him and then they will say, "You are a great man, and whatsoever you say is true. But we are helpless, poor dogs. We don't understand such big things." So all the dogs felt guilty because they couldn't stop. And they believed in the message of the leader, and he was right: rationally, they could follow. But what to do with the bodies? The bodies are irrational. Whenever there will be a chance — a sannyasin walking — they will bark: a policeman, a postman. . .because they are against uniforms.

It was almost impossible for them, and they had settled it that "That dog is a great man, and we cannot follow. He is like an *avatar* — something from the other shore. So we will worship him, but how can we follow him?" And that leader was always true to his word: he never barked. But one day everything failed. One night, dark night, the dogs decided that, "This great leader is always trying to convert us, and we never listen to him. At least once a year, on the birthday of the leader, we should keep complete fast: no barking—absolute silence —no matter how difficult. At least once a year we can do that," they decided.

And on that night not a single dog barked. The leader went from this corner to that, this street to that, to watch, because wherever dogs will be barking, he will preach. He started feeling very miserable because nobody is barking; the whole night completely silent, as if no dog exists. . . He went many places, watched, and by the midnight it was so impossible for him that he moved in a dark corner and barked!

The moment the other dogs heard that one has broken, they said, "Now there is no problem." They didn't know that the leader has done it. They thought one of them has broken the vow. But now it was impossible for them to contain; the whole city barked. The leader came out and he started preaching!

This will be the condition of your social revolutionaries, reformers, Gandhians, Marxians and others—all brands. They will be in such a difficulty if the world is really changed. If the world fulfills really the utopia of their minds and imaginations, they will commit suicide or they will go mad. Or they will start preaching just opposite, just the contradictory, just the opposite whatsoever they are preaching now.

They come to me and they say, "How you can tell people to be silent when the world is in such a misery?" They think first the misery has to be removed, then people will be silent? No, if people are silent misery can be removed, because only silence can remove the misery. Misery is an attitude. It is less concerned with material conditions, more concerned with the inner mind, the inner consciousness. Even a poor man can be happy, and once he is happy many things start falling in line.

Soon he may not be a poor man, because how can you be poor when you are happy? When you are happy, the whole world participates with you. When you are unhappy, everything goes wrong. You create all around a situation which helps your unhappiness to be there. This is the dynamics of the mind. It is a self-defeating system. You feel miserable, then more misery attracts towards you. When more misery attracts you say, "How I can be silent? So much misery there." Then even more misery is attracted toward you. Then you say, "It is impossible now. And those who say they are happy must be telling lies: these Buddhas, Krishnas, they must be telling lies. These Patanjalis, they must be liars, because it is possible, so much misery?"

Then you are in a self-defeating system. You attract, and not only you attract for yourself: when one person is miserable, he helps others also to be miserable, because they are also fools like you. Seeing you in misery, they sympathize. When they sympathize, they become vulnerable. So it is just like that: one ill person infects the whole community.

Mulla Nasruddin's doctor sent him a bill. It was too much. His child was ill: Nasruddin's small son was ill. He phoned to the doctor that "This is too much." The doctor said, "But I had to come nine times to see your son, so that has to be accounted for." Nasruddin said, "And don't forget that my son infected the whole village, and you have been earning a lot. In fact you should pay me something."

When one person is miserable, he infects. Misery is infectious just as happiness is infectious. And if you are vulnerable towards misery — as you are because you are always seeking unknowingly — your mind seeks misery, because with misery you feel sympathy; with happiness you feel jealous.

Mulla Nasruddin's wife told me once that "If you are

going to New Delhi—the winter is coming—you bring me a drop-dead coat." I was surprised. I couldn't follow what she means. I told her anyway, "I don't know much about coats, but I have never heard. What is a drop-dead coat?" She said, "You never heard?" and started laughing and said, "A drop-dead coat is a coat, when you put it on, neighbors drop dead!"

Unless others drop dead, you don't feel alive. Unless others are in misery, you don't feel happy. But how can you feel happy when others are unhappy, and how can you feel alive really when others are dead? We exist together. And sometimes you may be the cause of many people's misery. Then you are earning a karma. You may not have directly hit them; you may not have been violent to them. Subtle is the law! You need not be a murderer, but if simply you infect people by your misery, you are participating in it; you are creating misery. And you are responsible for it, and you will have to pay for it. Very subtle is the mechanism!

Just two, three days before it happened a sannyasin attacked Laxmi. You may not have observed that you all are responsible for it, because many of you have been feeling antagonism towards Laxmi. That sannyasin is just a victim, just the weakest link among you. He has expressed your antagonism, that's all, and he was the weakest; he became the victim, and now you will feel that he is responsible. That's not true. You participated. Subtle is the law!

How you participated? Deep down, whenever somebody managing—and Laxmi is managing things around here. . . There are many situations in which you will feel antagonistic, in which she will have to say no to you, in which you will feel hurt—it cannot be avoided —in which you feel that enough attention is not being paid to you, in which you feel that you are treated as if you are nobody. Your ego feels hurt and you feel antagonism.

If many people feel antagonism towards a person,

then the weakest amongst them will become the victim;
he will do something. He was the craziest amongst you,
that's right. But he alone is not responsible. If you have
ever felt antagonism towards Laxmi, that is part and
you have earned a karma, and unless you become so
subtly aware you cannot become enlightened. Things
are very complicated.

Now in the West also, psychoanalysts have found
that the whole family is responsible if one person goes
mad—whole family! Now they think that the family has
to be treated, not one person, because when one person
goes mad that only shows that the whole family has
inner tensions. This is the weakest of them all, so immediately he shows the whole thing, he becomes the ex-
pression of the whole family, and if you treat him it
won't help. In the hospital he may be okay: back home
he will fall ill again because the whole family has inner
tensions and this is the weakest.

Children suffer too much because of parents. They
are fighting; they are always creating anxiety and tension around the house. The whole house exists not as a
peaceful community, but as an inner war and conflict.
The child is vulnerable more; the child starts behaving
in eccentric ways—now you have an excuse that you are
tense and worried because of the child. And now the
father and mother both can be concerned with the child;
they will take him to the psychoanalyst and the doctor,
and they can forget their own conflict.

And this child becomes a cementing force, if he is ill;
then they have to pay more attention to him. And now
they have an excuse why they are worried and tense and
in anguish—because the child is ill—and they don't
know just the reverse is the case. . .*because* they are
worried, tense in conflict. The child is innocent, tender;
he can be affected immediately, he has no protection
around him yet. And if the child becomes really healthy,
the parents will be in more difficulty—because then
there is no excuse.

This is a community; you live here as a family. Many tensions are bound to be there, be aware. Be alert about those tensions because your tensions can create a force. They can become accumulative, and suddenly some-body who is weak, vulnerable, simple, may become the shelter of the accumulated force, and then he reacts in a way. Then you all can throw the responsibility on him. But that is not true if you ever have felt any antagonism, you are part of it. And the same is true in the greater world also.

When Godase murdered Gandhi, I never said that Godase is responsible. He was the weakest link; that is true. But the whole Hindu mind was responsible, deep currents of Hindu antagonism against Gandhi. The feel-ing that he is for Moslems, Mohammedans, was accu-mulating. This is an actual phenomenon: antagonism becomes accumulated. Just like a cloud, it hovers, and then somewhere a weak heart, a very unprotected man, becomes the victim. The cloud gets roots into him and then the explosion. And then everybody is freed: Go-dase is responsible—murdering Gandhi—so you can kill Godase and be finished. Then the whole country moves in the same way, and the Hindu mind remains the same: no change. Subtle is the law!

Always find the dynamics of mind. Only then you will be transformed; otherwise not.

*The mind becomes tranquil by cultivating*
*attitudes of friendliness towards the happy,*
*compassion towards the miserable, joy towards*
*the virtuous. . .*

Look! Patanjali is making steps—and beautiful and very subtle, but exactly scientific.

*. . .joy towards the virtuous, and indifference*
*towards the evil.*

When you feel somebody is a virtuous man, *joy*, the ordinary attitude is that he must be deceiving. How anybody can be more virtuous than you? Hence so much criticism goes on.

Whenever there is somebody who is virtuous, you immediately start criticizing, you start finding faults with him. Somehow or other you have to bring him down. He cannot be virtuous. You cannot believe this. Patanjali says *joy*, because if you criticize a virtuous man, deep down you are criticizing virtue. If you criticize a virtuous man, you are coming to a point to believe that virtue is impossible in this world. Then you will feel at ease. Then you can move on your evil ways easily because, "Nobody is virtuous; everybody is just like me—even worse than me." That's why so much condemnation goes on—criticism, condemnation.

If somebody says, "That person is a very beautiful person," you immediately find something to criticize. You cannot tolerate—because if somebody is virtuous and you are not, your ego is shattered, and then you start feeling that "I have to change myself," which is an arduous effort. The simple is to condemn; the simple is to criticize; the simple is to say, "No! Prove! What are you saying? First, prove how he is virtuous!" And it is difficult to prove virtue; it is very easy to unprove anything. It is very difficult to prove!

One of the greatest Russian storytellers is Turgenev. He has written a story. The story is that in a small village a man was thought to be stupid, and he was. And the whole town laughed at him. He was just like a fool, and everybody in the town enjoyed his foolishness. But he was tired of his foolishness, so he asked a wise man, "What to do?"

The wise man said, "Nothing! Simply, whenever somebody is praising somebody, you condemn. Somebody is saying that 'That man is a saint,' immediately say, 'No! I know well he is a sinner!' Somebody says, 'This book is very great,' immediately say, 'I have read it and studied it.' Don't bother whether you have read it or not; simply say, 'This is rubbish.' If somebody is saying, 'This painting is one of the greatest works of art,' simply say, 'But what it is? — just a canvas and colors. A child can do it!' Criticize, say no, ask for proofs, and after seven days come to me."

Within seven days the town started feeling that this man is a genius: "We never knew about his talents, and he is such a genius about everything. You show him a painting and he shows the faults. You show him a great book, and he shows the faults. He is such a great critical mind! An analyst! A genius!"

Seventh day he came to the wise man and he said, "Now there is no need to take any advice from you. You are a fool!" The whole town used to believe in that sage, and they all said that "Our genius has said that he is a fool; he must be."

People always believe in the negative easily because to disprove a no is very difficult — how can you prove? How can you prove that Jesus is son of God? How you will prove? Two thousand years, and Christian theology has been proving without proving it. But within seconds it was proved that he was a sinner, a vagabond, and they killed — within seconds! Somebody said that "I have seen this man coming out of a prostitute's house" — finished! Nobody bothers whether this man who is saying that "I have seen," is believable or not — nobody bothers! The negative is always believed easily because it is also helping your ego. The positive is not believed.

You can say no whenever there is virtue. But you are not harming the virtuous man: you are harming you. You are self-destructive. You are, in fact, committing suicide slowly — poisoning yourself. When you say that "This man is not virtuous, that man is not virtuous," what are you, in fact, creating? You are creating a milieu in which you will come to believe that virtue is impossible; and when virtue is impossible, there is no need to attempt. Then you fall down. Then you settle wherever you are. Growth becomes impossible. And you would like to settle, but then you settle in misery because you are miserable.

You all have settled completely. This settlement has to be broken; you have to be unsettled. Wherever you are you have to be uprooted and replanted in a higher plane, and that is possible only if you are joyful towards the virtuous.

> . . .joy towards the virtuous and indifference towards the evil.

Don't even condemn evil.

The temptation is there; you would like to condemn even virtue. And Patanjali says don't condemn evil. Why? He knows the inner dynamics of the mind: because if you too much condemn evil, you pay too much attention to evil, and by and by, you become attuned to it. If you say that "This is wrong, that is wrong," you are paying too much attention to the wrong. You will become addicted with the wrong. If you pay too much attention to anything, you become hypnotized. And whatsoever you are condemning you will commit, because it will become an attraction, a deep-down attraction. Otherwise, why bother? They are sinners, but who are you to bother about them?

Jesus says, "Judge ye not. . ." That's what Patanjali means—indifference; don't judge this way or that—be indifferent. Don't say yes or no; don't condemn, don't appreciate. Simply leave it to the divine; it is none of your business. A man is a thief: it is his business. It is his and God's. Let them settle themselves; you don't come in. Who is asking you to come in? Jesus says, "Judge ye not. . ." Patanjali says, "Be indifferent."

One of the greatest hypnotists of the world, Emile Coué, discovered a law—law of hypnosis. He called it the Law of Reverse Effect. If you are too much against something, you will become a victim. See a new person learning bicycle on the road. The road is sixty feet wide, and there is a milestone by the side of the road. Even if you are a perfect cyclist and you make the target of the stone that "I will go and crash with the stone," sometimes you may miss. But never the new learner — never! He never misses the cornerstone. In a subtle way, his cycle moves towards the stone, and sixty feet wide is the road! Even with blindfolded eyes you can move on it — even if there is nobody on the road, it is completely silent, nobody is moving. . .

What happens to this new learner? A law is working. Emile Coué calls it the Law of the Reverse Effect. Immediately, because he is a learner, he is afraid, so he looks around, where is the fear point — where he can go wrong? The whole road is okay, but this stone, this red stone by the corner, that is the danger: "I may crash with it." Now there is an affinity created. Now his attention is towards the stone; the whole road is forgotten. And he is a learner! His hands tremble, and he is looking at the stone, and by and by he feels that the cycle is moving. Once he feels the cycle. . .

The cycle has to follow your attention: cycle has no will of its own. It follows you wherever you are going, and you follow your eyes, and eyes follow a subtle hypnosis, an attentiveness. You are looking at the stone, the hands move that way. You become more and more afraid. The more you are afraid, the more caught, because now the stone seems to be an evil force, as if the stone is attracting you. The whole road is forgotten, the cycle is forgotten, the learner is forgotten. Only the stone is there; you are hypnotized. You will go and crash with the stone. Now you have fulfilled your mind; next time you will be more afraid. Now where to break out of it?

When you say that something is wrong, go in the monasteries — the monks condemning sex. Sex has become the milestone. Twenty-four hours they are thinking about it: trying to avoid it is thinking about it. The more you try to avoid it, the more you are hypnotized.

That is why in the old scriptures it is said whenever a saint concentrates, beautiful girls from heaven come and try to disturb his mind. Why beautiful girls should be interested? Somebody is sitting under a tree with closed eyes, why beautiful girls will be interested in this man?

Nobody comes from anywhere, but he is so much against sex it becomes a hypnosis. He is so much hypnotized that now dreams become real. He opens the eyes and sees a beautiful naked girl standing there. You need a pornographic book to see a nude woman. If you go to the monastery you will not need a pornographic book: you create your pornography yourself all around. And then the seer, the man who was concentrating, becomes more afraid: he closes his eyes, clenches his fist. Now inside the woman is standing.

And you cannot find such beautiful women on this earth because they are creations of dream — hypnosis byproducts — and the more he becomes afraid, the more they are there. They will rub with his body, they will touch his head, they will cling and embrace him. He is completely mad, but this happens. This is happening to you also. Degrees may differ, but this is what is happening. Whatsoever you are against, you will be joined with it deep down.

Never be against anything. To be against evil is to fall a victim. Then you are falling in the hands of the evil. Indifference: if you follow indifference, it means it is none of your concern. Somebody is stealing: that is his karma. He will know and he will have to suffer. That is not your business at all: you don't think about it, don't pay any attention to it. There is a prostitute: she is selling her body — that is her business. You don't have condemnation in you, otherwise you will be attracted towards her.

It happened — a very old story — that a saint and a prostitute lived together. They were neighbors, and then they died. The saint was very famous. Death came and started trying to take the saint to the hell. And they died on the same day, the prostitute also.

The saint was surprised because the prostitute was taken on the road towards heaven. So he said, "What is this? There seems some misunderstanding. I am the one who should be led towards heaven. And this is a prostitute!"

Death said, "We know, but now if you want, we can explain you: there is no misunderstanding. There are the orders — that the prostitute has to be brought to heaven and the saint has to be thrown into hell." The saint said, "But why?" Even the prostitute could not believe. She said, "Something must be wrong. I must be thrown in heaven? And he is a saint — a great saint. We worshipped him. Take him to heaven."

Death said, "No, that's not possible, because he was a saint just on the surface, and he was thinking continuously of you. And when you will sing in the night, he will come and listen to you. He will stand just near the fence and listen to you. And millions of times he would like to go to see you, love you; millions of times he dreamed of you. He was continuously thinking about you. On the lips was the name of God; in the heart was the image of you."

And the same from the opposite direction was true with the prostitute. She was selling her body, but always thinking that she would like to have a life like this saint who lives in a temple. "How pure he is!" She dreamt about the saint, the purity, the saintliness, the virtue that she is missing. And when customers would have gone, she will pray to God that "Next time don't make me a prostitute again. Make me a worshipper; make me a meditator. I would like to serve in the temple."

And many times she thought to go into the temple, but thinking that she is so much in sin, it was not good to enter the temple: "The place is so holy and I am such a sinner." And many times she wanted to touch the feet of the saint, but thinking that that will not be good: "I am not worthy enough to touch his feet." So when the saint will pass, she will just collect the dust on the road from where the saint has passed, and she will worship that dust.

What you are outwardly is not the question. What is your inner hypnosis will decide your future course of life. Be indifferent to evil. Indifference does not mean apathy—remember. These are subtle distinctions. Indifference doesn't mean apathy! It does not mean that close your eyes, because even if you close you have taken a standpoint, attitude. It does not mean don't bother, because there also is a subtle condemnation. Indifference simply means as if it doesn't exist, as if it is not there. No attitude indifference means. You pass as if it is not happening.

*Upeksha*, the word Patanjali uses, is very beautiful. It is neither apathy nor antagonism nor escape. It is simple indifference without any attitude—remember, without any attitude, because you can be indifferent with an attitude. You can think it is not worth—it is not worthy of me to think about it. No, then you have an attitude, and a subtle condemnation is hidden in it. Indifference means simply, "Who are you to decide, to judge?" You think about you, "Who are you? How can you say what is evil and what is good? Who knows?"

Because life is such a complexity the evil becomes good, the good becomes evil—they change. Sinners have been known to reach the ultimate; saints have been known to be thrown into hell. So who knows? And who are you? Who is asking you? You take care of yourself. Even if you can do that, enough you have done. You be more mindful and aware; then an indifference comes to you without any attitude.

It happened: Vivekananda, before he went to America and became a world-famous figure, stayed in Jaipur Maharaja's palace. The Maharaja was a lover of Vivekananda and Ramakrishna. As maharajas go, when

Vivekananda came to stay in his palace he made a great festival out of it, and he called prostitutes to dance and sing in reception. . .as maharajas go: they have their own minds. He completely forgot that to receive a sannyasin with the singing of prostitutes and dancing of prostitutes doesn't suit. But he couldn't know anything else. He always knew that when you have to receive somebody, drinking, dancing has to be done.

And Vivekananda was still immature; he was not a perfect sannyasin yet. Had he been a perfect sannyasin, then there was indifference—no problem—but he was not indifferent yet. He has not gone that deep into Patanjali even. He was a young man, and a very suppressive one who was suppressing his sex and everything. When he saw the prostitutes, he simply locked his room and would not come out of it.

The Maharaja came and he asked his forgiveness. He said, "We don't know. We have never received any sannyasin. We always receive kings, so we know the ways. So we are sorry, but now it will be too much insulting, because this is the greatest prostitute in the country—and very costly. And we have paid, and to say her to move and go will be insulting to her, and if you don't come she will feel very much hurt. So come out."

But Vivekananda was afraid to come out; that's why I say he was still immature, still not a seasoned sannyasin. Still indifference is not there—a condemnation: "A prostitute?"—he was very angry, and he said, "No!" Then the prostitute started singing without him, and she sang a song of a saint. The song is very beautiful. The song says that "I know that I am not worthy of you, but you could have been a little more compassionate. I am dirt on the road; that I know. But you need not be so antagonistic to me. I am nobody—ignorant, a sinner. But you are a saint; why are you afraid of me?"

It is said Vivekananda heard from his room. The prostitute was weeping and singing, and he felt—he felt the whole situation of what he is doing. It is immature, childish. Why he is afraid? Fear exists only if you are attracted. You will be afraid of women if you are attracted of women. If you are not attracted, the fear disappears. What is the fear? An indifference comes without any antagonism.

He opened the door: he couldn't contain himself; he was defeated by the prostitute. The prostitute became victorious; he had to come out. He came and he sat, and he wrote in his diary that "A new revelation has been given to me by the divine. I was afraid. . .must be some lust within me. That's why I was afraid. But the woman defeated me completely, and I have never seen such a pure soul. The tears were so innocent and the singing and the dancing were so holy that I would have missed. And sitting near her, for the first time I became aware that it is not a question who is there outside; it is a question what is."

That night he wrote in his diary that "Now I can even sleep with that woman in the bed and there will be no fear." He transcended. That prostitute helped him to transcend. This is a miracle. Ramakrishna couldn't help, and a prostitute helped him. So nobody knows from where the help will come. Nobody knows what is evil and what is good. Who can decide? Mind is impotent and helpless. So don't take any attitude: that is the meaning of being indifferent.

*The mind also becomes tranquil by alternately expelling and retaining the breath.*

Patanjali gives other alternatives also. If you can do this —being happy with happy people, friendly; compassion with the miserable, joy with the virtuous, indifference with the evil ones—if you can do this, then you enter from the transformation of the mind towards the supermind. If you cannot do—because it is difficult, not easy —then there are other ways. Don't feel depressed.

Says Patanjali:

*The mind also becomes tranquil by alternately expelling and retaining the breath.*

Then you enter through the physiology. This is entering through the mind—the first: the second is entering through the physiology.

Breathing and thinking are deeply connected, as if they are two poles of one thing. You also sometimes become aware, if you are a little mindful, that whenever the mind changes, the breathing changes. For example, you are angry: immediately the breathing changes, the rhythm is gone. The breathing has a different quality. It is non-rhythmic.

When you have passion, lust, sex takes over, the breathing changes; it becomes feverish, mad. When you are silent, just not doing anything, just feeling very relaxed, the breathing has a different rhythm. If you watch, and Patanjali must have watched very deeply. . .he says if you watch deeply you can find what type of breathing and its rhythm creates what type of mind. If you feel friendly, the breathing is different. If you feel antagonistic, angry, the breathing is different. So either change the mind and the breathing will change, or you can do the opposite: change the breathing and the mind will change. Change the rhythm of breathing, and the mind will immediately change.

When you feel happy, silent, joyous, remember the rhythm of the breathing. Next time when anger comes, you don't allow the breathing to change; you retain the rhythm of breathing as if you are happy. Anger is not possible then because the breathing creates the situation. The breathing forces the inner glands in the body which release chemicals in the blood.

That's why you become red when you are angry: certain chemicals have come into the blood, and you become feverish. Your temperature goes high. The body is ready to fight or take flight; the body is in an emergency. Through hammering of the breathing, this change comes.

Don't change the breathing. Just retain as if you are silent; just the breathing just has to follow a silent pattern — you will feel it impossible to become angry. When you are feeling very passionate, lust, sex takes over. Just try to be tranquil in the breathing, and you feel sex has disappeared.

Here he suggests a method:

*The mind also becomes tranquil by alternately expelling and retaining the breath.*

You can do two things: whenever you feel the mind is not tranquil — tense, worried, chattering, anxiety, constantly dreaming — do one thing: first exhale deeply. Always start by exhaling. Exhale deeply: as much as you can, throw the air out. With the throwing of the air the mood will be thrown out, because breathing is everything.

And then expel the breath as far as possible. Take the belly in and retain for few seconds; don't inhale. Let the air be out, and you don't inhale for few seconds. Then allow the body to inhale. Inhale deeply — as much as you can. Again stop for few seconds. The same should be the gap as you retain the breath out — if you retain for three seconds, retain the breath in three seconds. Throw it out; retain for three seconds. Take in; retain for three seconds. But it has to be thrown out completely. Exhale totally and inhale totally, and make a rhythm. Retain, in; retain, out. Retain, in; retain, out. Immediately you will feel a change coming into your whole being. The mood is gone. A new climate has entered into you.

What happens? Why is it so? For many reaons: one, when you start creating this rhythm, your mind is completely diverted. You cannot be angry, because a new thing has started, and mind cannot have two things together. Your mind is now filled with exhaling, inhaling, retaining, creating a rhythm. You are completely absorbed in it, the cooperation with anger is broken: one thing.

This exhaling, inhaling, cleanses the whole body. When you exhale out and retain for three seconds or five seconds — as much as you want, as much as you can — what happens inside? The whole body throws all that is poisonous into the blood. Air is out and the body gets a gap. In that gap all the poisons are thrown out. They come to the heart, they accumulate there — poisonous gases, nitrogen, carbon dioxide, they all gather together there.

You don't give a chance for them to gather together. You go on breathing in and out. There is no gap, no pause. In that pause, a gap is created, an emptiness. In that emptiness, everything flows and fills it. Then you take a deep inhalation and then you retain. All those poisonous gases become mixed with the breathing; then you again exhale and throw them out. Again pause. Let the poisons gather. And this is a way of throwing things out.

Mind and breath are so much connected — have to be, because breathing is life. A man can be without mind, but cannot be without breathing. Breathing is deeper than mind. Your brain can be operated completely; you will be alive if you can breathe. If the breathing continues, you will be alive. The brain can be taken out completely. You will vegetate, but you will be alive. You will not be able to open the eyes and talk or do anything, but on the bed you can be alive, vegetating for many years. But mind cannot! If the breathing stops, mind disappears.

Yoga found this basic thing — that breathing is deeper than thinking. If you change breathing, you change thinking. And once you know the key, that breathing has the key, you can create any climate that you want: it is up to you. The way you breathe it depends on it. Just you do one thing: for seven days, you just make a notebook of the different types of breathing that happen with different moods. You are angry: take a notebook and just count breathing — how much you inhale and how much you exhale. Five counts you inhale, three counts you exhale — note it down.

Sometime you are feeling very, very beautiful — note it down, what is the proportion of inhalation and exhalation, what is the length, is there any pause — note it down. And for seven days just make a diary to feel your own breathing, how it is connected with your moods. Then you can sort it out. Then whenever you want to drop a mood, just use the opposite pattern. Or, if you want to bring a mood, then use the pattern.

Actors, knowingly, unknowingly, come to know it because sometimes they have to be angry without being angry. So what they will do? They will have to create the breathing pattern. They may not be aware, but they will start breathing as if they are angry, and soon the blood rushes in and poisons are released. And without being angry their eyes are red, and they are in a subtle anger state without being angry. They have to make love without being in love; they have to show love without being in love. How they do it? They know a certain secret of yoga.

That's why I always say a yogi can become the most perfect actor. He is! His stage is vast, that's all. He is acting — not acting on the stage, but on the stage of the world. He is an actor; he is not a doer. And the difference is that he is taking part in a great drama and he can remain a witness to it and he can remain aloof and detached.

*When meditation produces extraordinary sense perceptions, the mind gains confidence and this helps perseverance.*

If you work out your breathing pattern, and you find the secret keys how to change the climate of the mind, how to change the moods. . . And if you work from both the poles, that will be better. And try to be friendly towards happy, indifferent towards the evil, and continue the change and transformation of your breathing patterns also. Then there will be extraordinary sense perceptions.

If you have taken LSD, marijuana, hashish, then you know extraordinary sense perceptions happen. You look ordinary things, and they become extraordinary. Aldous Huxley remembers that when he took for the first time LSD he was sitting before an ordinary chair, and when he became more and more deep with the drug, when he was on, the chair immediately started changing color. Radiant it became: an ordinary chair — he had never paid any attention to it — became so beautiful, many colors coming out of it, as if it is made of diamonds. Such beautiful shapes and nuances that he couldn't believe his eyes, what is happening. Later on he remembered this must have happened to Van Gogh, because he has painted a chair almost exactly the same.

A poet need not take LSD. He has an inbuilt system of throwing LSD in the body. That is the difference between a poet and an ordinary man. That's why they say a poet is born, not made: because he has an extraordinary body structure. The chemicals in his body have a different quantity and quality to them. That's why where you don't see anything he sees miracles. You see an ordinary tree, and he sees something unbelievable. You see ordinary clouds: a poet, if he is really a poet, never sees anything ordinary; everything is extraordinarily beautiful.

The same happens to a yogi: because when you change your breathing and your attitudes, your body chemistry changes its pattern; you are going through a chemical transformation, and then your eyes become clear, a new perceptivity happens. The old same tree becomes absolutely new. You never knew the shade of its green: it becomes radiant. The whole world all around you takes a new shape. It is a paradise now — not the ordinary old rotten earth.

People around you are no more the same. Your ordinary wife becomes a most beautiful woman. Everything

changes with your clarity of perception. When your
eyes change, everything changes. Says Patanjali,

> *When meditation produces extraordinary sense*
> *perceptions, the mind gains confidence and that*
> *helps perseverance.*

Then you become confident that you are on the right
path. The world is becoming more and more beautiful;
the ugliness is disappearing. The world is becoming
more and more a harmony; the discord is disappearing.
The world is becoming more and more home; you are
feeling more and more at ease in it. It is friendly. It is a
love affair with you and the universe. You become more
confident, and more perseverance comes to your effort.

> *Also, meditate on the inner light which is*
> *serene, beyond all sorrow.*

This can be done only when you have attained a certain
quality of perceptivity. Then you can close the eyes and
you can find a flame — a beautiful flame near the heart, a
blue light. But right now you cannot see it. It is there; it
has been always there. When you die, that blue light
goes out of your body. But you cannot see it because
when you were alive you couldn't see it.

And others will also be not able to see it, that something is going out; but Kirlian in Soviet Russia, he has
taken photographs with very sensitive films. When a
person dies, something happens around. Some body-
energy, some light-like thing, leaves, goes and disappears into the cosmos. That light is always there: that is
your center of being. It is near the heart — with a blue
flame.

When you have some perception, you can see the
beautiful world all around you — when your eyes are
clear. You close them and you move nearer the heart;
you try to find what is there. First you will feel darkness. It is just like as you come from the outside on a hot
sunny day inside the room, and you feel everything is

dark. But wait! Let the eyes be attuned with the darkness, and soon you start seeing things in the house.

You have been outside for millions of lives. When for the first time you come in, nothing is there except darkness, emptiness. But wait! It will take few days – even few months, but just wait, close the eyes and look down in the heart. Suddenly, one day it happens: you see a light, a flame. Then concentrate on that flame.

Nothing is more blissful than that. Nothing is more dancing, singing, musical, harmonious like that inner blue light within your heart. And the more you concentrate, the more you become tranquil, silent, calm, collected. then there is no darkness for you. When your heart is filled with light, the whole universe is filled with light.

*Also, meditate on the inner light which is serene and beyond all sorrow.*

*Also, meditate on one who has attained desirelessness.*

That too! All alternatives Patanjali is giving you! A *veetaraga*, one who has gone beyond all desires – also meditate on him. Mahavira, Buddha, Patanjali – your own – Zarathustra, Mohammed, Christ or anybody you feel an affinity and love. . . Meditate on one who has gone beyond desires. Meditate on your Master, on your guru, who has gone beyond desires. How it will help? It helps, because when you meditate on someone who has gone beyond desires he becomes a magnetic force in you. You allow him to enter within you; he pulls you out of yourself. This becomes your availability to him.

If you meditate on someone who has gone beyond desires, you will become like him sooner or later, because meditation makes you like the object of meditation itself. If you meditate on money, you will become just like money. Go and look at a miser; he has no more a soul. He has only a bank balance; he has nothing inside. If you listen, you will just hear notes, rupees: you will not find any heart there. Whatsoever you pay your attention, you become like it. So be aware. Don't pay attention to something you would not like to become. Only pay attention to something you would like to become, because this is the beginning. The seed is sown with the attention, and soon it will become a tree.

You sow the seeds of hell, and when it becomes a tree then you say, "Why I am so miserable?" You always pay attention to the wrong; you always look to that which is negative. You always pay attention to the fault; then you become faulty.

Don't pay attention to the fault. Pay attention to the beautiful. Why count the thorns? Why not see the flower? Why count the nights? Why not count the days? If you count the nights, then there are two nights and only one day between the two. If you count the days, then there are two days and only one night in between. And it makes a lot of difference. Look at the light side if you want to become light; look at the dark if you want to become dark.

Says Patanjali:

*Also, meditate on one who has attained desirelessness.*

Seek a Master; surrender to a Master. Be attentive to him. Listen, watch, eat and drink him. Let him enter you; allow your heart to be filled with him. Soon you will be on a journey, because the object of attention ultimately becomes the goal of your life. And attention is a secret relationship. Through attention you become the object of your attention.

Krishnamurti goes on saying, "The observer becomes the observed." He is right: whatsoever you observe, you will become. So be alert! Beware! Don't observe something which you would not like to become, because that is your goal; you are sowing the seeds

Live near a *veetaraga* — a man who is beyond desires. Live near a man who has no more to fulfill here, who is fulfilled. His very fulfilledness will overflood you, and he will become a catalyst.

He will not do anything, because a man who is beyond desires cannot do anything. Even he cannot help you because help is also a desire. Much help comes through him, but he doesn't help you. He becomes a catalyst without doing anything, if you allow him; he drops into your heart and his very presence crystallizes you.

The Alpha

Alpha

Is

The

Omega

The first question:

*Do positive thoughts bring happenings too?—*
*like wishing for enlightenment.*

THAT IS TOO MUCH ASKING from positive thoughts because enlightenment is beyond duality: it is neither negative nor positive. When both the polarities are dropped, it happens. With positive thoughts many things are possible —not enlightenment.

You can be happy, but not blissful. Happiness comes and goes; the opposite always exists with it. When you are happy, just by the side of happiness unhappiness is waiting for its own time. It is standing in the queue. When you are loving, it is positive; hate is waiting for its own time.

Positive cannot go beyond duality. It is good as far as it goes, but to ask enlightenment from it is too much. Never expect that. Negative has to be dropped to attain to the positive. Positive has also to be dropped to attain to the beyond. First drop the negative, then drop the positive; then nothing is left. That nothingness is enlightenment; then there is no more mind.

Mind is either negative or positive, happy, unhappy, loving, hateful; anger, compassion, day and night, birth and death — all belong to mind. But *you* don't belong to mind. You are beyond it — encased in the mind, but beyond it.

Enlightenment is not of the mind. It is of you. The realization that "I am not the mind" is enlightenment. If you remain negative you remain in the valley part of the mind. If you are positive, you attain to the peak part of the mind. But neither transcends the mental plane of your being: drop both.

It is difficult to drop the positive. It is easy to drop the negative because the negative gives you misery. It is a hell; you can drop it. But look at the misfortune: you have not even dropped that. You cling to the negative also. You cling to misery as if it is a treasure. You cling to your unhappiness just because it has become an old habit, and you need something to cling. Not finding anything, you cling to your hell. But, remember, to drop the negative is easy, howsoever difficult it seems. Compared to the positive it is very easy because it is misery.

To drop the positive means to drop the happiness; to drop the positive means to drop all that looks like flowers, all that is beautiful. The negative is the ugly, positive is the beautiful. The negative is death, positive is life. But if you can drop the negative. . .so take the first step. First feel the misery, how much misery is given by the negative to you. Just watch how misery arises out of it: just watch and feel. The very feeling that the negative is creating misery will become the dropping.

But mind has a very deep trick. Whenever you are miserable, it always says somebody else is responsible. Be alert, because if you are a victim of this trick then the negative can never be dropped. This is how the negative is hiding itself. You are angry. The mind says somebody has insulted and that's why you are angry — that is not right. Somebody may have insulted, but that is just an excuse. You were already waiting to be angry. Anger was accumulating within you, otherwise somebody would have insulted — there would have been no anger.

The insult may become the visible cause of it, but it is not really the cause. You are boiling within. In fact, the person who insults you helps you. He helps you to bring your inner turmoil out and be finished with it. You are in such a bad shape that even insult helps you. The enemy helps you because he helps you to bring all negativity out. At least you are unburdened for a time being.

Mind has this trick always to divert your consciousness towards the other. Immediately something goes wrong and you start looking who has done this. In that looking you miss, and the real culprit is hiding behind.

Make it an absolute law that whenever something is wrong, immediately close the eyes and look for the real culprit. And you will be able to see because it is a truth. It is a reality. It is true that you accumulate anger; that's why you become angry. It is true that you accumulate hate; that's why you feel hatred. The other is not a real cause. In Sanskrit, they have two terms. One term is *karan* — the real cause, and another term is *nimitta* — the unreal cause. And the *nimitta*, the unreal cause which appears as cause but is not the cause, befools you. It has been befooling you for many, many lives.

Immediately close the eyes and go in whenever you feel something miserable happening, because that is the right moment to catch the culprit redhanded. Otherwise you will not be able to catch it. When the anger has disappeared, you will close the eyes. You will not find anything there. In a red-hot situation, don't miss the point. Make it a meditation.

And if you start feeling no need is there for any method to drop the negative. . . Negative is so ugly, it is such a disease — how you are carrying it is amazing. Dropping is nothing; carrying is amazing. It has riddled all the Buddhas — how you carry and why you carry all of your diseases so lovingly? You are so careful about them; you protect all that is wrong. Protected, it gets deeper and deeper roots in you.

Once realized that this is my own negativity which creates the problem, it falls by itself. And then there is a beauty, when the negative mind falls by itself. If you try to drop it, it will cling—because the very effort to drop it shows that your understanding is not mature. All renunciation is immaturity; you are not ripe for it. That's why effort is needed to drop it. I am carrying rubbish; do I need any effort to drop it, except the understanding that this is rubbish? If I need any effort to drop it, that means I am supplementing my understanding with effort. Understanding itself is not enough; that's why effort is needed.

All those who have known, they say effort is needed because your understanding is not there. It may be an intellectual thing, but really you have not felt the situation, otherwise you simply drop it. A snake passes the path; you simply jump. There is no effort in the jump. You don't decide to jump; you don't make a logical syllogism within you that "There is a snake, and wherever there is a snake there is danger; hence, I must jump." You don't make a logical step-by-step syllogism. Even Aristotle will jump. Later on he can make the syllogism, but right now, when the snake is there, the snake doesn't bother about your logic, and the whole situation is so dangerous. . .the very understanding that the situation is dangerous is enough.

For the negative to drop, no effort is needed—only understanding. Then arises the real problem: how to drop the positive—because it is so beautiful. And for you who have not known the beyond, it is the ultimate in happiness—so happy. Look at a couple in love; look at their eyes, the way they walk hand in each other's hand: they are happy. Tell them to drop this positive mind and they will think, "Are you crazy?" For this they have been waiting and now it has happened. And here comes a Buddha and says, "Drop it."

When somebody is succeeding, reaching higher and higher on the ladder, tell him to drop it. That is his very purpose, in his eyes. And if he even thinks to drop it, he knows he will drop in misery.

Because from the positive where you will move? — you know only two possibilities: positive or negative. If you drop the positive, you move to the negative. That's why negative has to be dropped first: so there is nothing to move to the negative. Otherwise, if you drop the positive, immediately the negative enters. If you are not happy, then what you will be? — unhappy! If you are not silent, what you will be? — a chatterbox! Hence, drop the negative first so one alternative is closed — you cannot move that way. Otherwise energy has a routine movement from positive to negative, from negative to positive. If the negative exists, there is every possibility the moment you drop the positive you will become the negative.

When you are not happy, you will be unhappy. You don't know that there is a third possibility also. That third possibility opens only when negative has been dropped and then you drop the positive. For a moment there will be a halt. Energy cannot move anywhere, not knowing where to move. The negative door is closed, the positive has been closed. You will be for a moment . . .and that moment will look like eternity. It will look very, very long — non-ending.

For a moment you will be just in the middle, not knowing what to do, where to go. This moment will look like madness. You are neither positive nor negative, then who you are? What is your identity? Your identity, name and form drop with the positive and negative. Suddenly you are nobody that you can recognize — just an energy phenomenon. And you cannot say how you are feeling. There is no feeling. If you can tolerate it, bear this moment, this is the greatest sacrifice, the greatest *tapascharya,* and the whole yoga prepares you for this moment. Otherwise the tendency will be to go somewhere, but don't remain in this vacuum. Be positive, be negative, but don't remain in this vacuum. You are nothing, as if you are disappearing. An abyss has opened, and you are falling into it.

At this moment a Master is needed who can say, "Wait! Don't be afraid; I am here." This is just a lie, but you need it. Nobody is there. Not even a Master can be there because the Master also ends when your mind ends. Now you are absolutely alone, but to be alone is so fearsome, so scary, so deathlike, that somebody is needed to give you courage. Because it is only a one moment's question and the lie helps.

And I tell you, all the Buddhas have been liars just because of compassion towards you. The Master says, "I am here. You don't worry; you go ahead." You gain confidence, you take the jump. Just a moment's question, and everything hangs there. The whole existence hangs there; the crossing point, the boiling point. If you take the step, you are lost to the mind forever. There will be no positive, no negative again.

You can be scared. You can again go back and enter into the negative or in the positive which is cozy, comfortable, familiar. You were entering into the unknown: this is the problem. First, the problem is how to drop the negative — a ripe understanding is needed — and which is the easiest, and you have not done even that.

Then the problem is how to drop the positive which is so beautiful and gives you such happiness. But if you drop the negative, if you become that much ripe, you will have a second understanding, a second transformation, in which you will be able to see that if you don't drop the positive, the negative will come back.

Then the positive loses its all positivity. It was positive only in comparison to the negative. Once the negative is thrown, even the positive becomes negative, because now you can see all this happiness is momentary. And when this moment is lost, where you will be? The negative will enter again.

Before the negative enters, drop it. Hell always comes through heaven. Heaven is just the gate; hell is the real place. Through heaven and the promise of heaven you enter hell. Hell is the real place; heaven is just the gate. Sooner or later—how can you remain at the gate forever?—you have to enter. Where you will go from the positive?

Once negative is dropped, you can see that positive is just the other aspect of it—not really contrary, not opposite, but a conspiracy. They are both in conspiracy; they are together. When this understanding arises, the positive has become the negative, you can drop it.

In fact, to say you can drop it is not good. It also drops. It has also become negative. Then you know that in this life there is nothing like happiness. Happiness is a trick of unhappiness to come in too. It is just like the egg and the hen relationship. What is a hen? It is the way of the egg to come back. And what is an egg? It is a way of the hen to come back.

Positive and negative are not real opposites. They are like hen and egg, mother and child. They help each other and come from each other. But this understanding is possible only when negative has been dropped. Then you can drop the positive also. And then you can stay in that transitory moment, which is the greatest moment in existence. You will never feel another moment so long— as if years are passing, because the vacuum. . . You lose all bearing; the whole past is lost, suddenly empty, not knowing where you are, who you are, what is happening.

This is the moment of madness. If you try to return from this moment, you will remain always mad. Many people go mad through meditation. From this moment they fall back, and now there is nothing to fall back to because the positive/negative has been dropped. They no more exist; the house is no more there. Once you leave the house it disappears. It depended on you; it is not a separate entity.

Mind is not a separate entity. It depends on you. Once you leave it, it is no more there. You cannot come back, fall back to it. That is the state of madness. You have not attained to the transcendence, and you come back and you look for the mind — it is no more there; the house has disappeared.

To be in this state is very, very painful. The real anguish for the first time happens. Hence, the Master — the need of the Master, who will not allow you to come back, who will force you to go ahead, because once you turn back it will take much effort to bring you again to that point. Maybe for many lives you may miss it because now there is no mind to understand even.

In Sufism this state is called the state of a *mast* — the state of a madman. This state is really difficult to understand because the man is and is not — both. He laughs and weeps together; he has lost all orientations. He does not know what is weeping and what is laughing. Is there any contradiction? He beats himself and enjoys, celebrates, beating himself. He does not know what he is doing, whether it is harmful or not harmful. He becomes completely dependent. He becomes like a small child; he has to be taken care of.

Without a Master, if somebody goes into meditation this can be the outcome. With a Master, the Master will be the barrier. He will be just standing behind you and he will not allow you to go back. He will become a rock. And finding no way to go back, you will have to take the jump. Nobody can take it for you. Nobody can be with you at that moment. But once you take this jump you have transcended all dualities. Negative, positive, both gone — and this is enlightenment.

I talk about the positive so that you can drop the negative. Once you drop the negative you are trapped. Then the positive has to be dropped. Each step leads to another in such a way that if you take the first step the second is bound to come. It is a chain. In fact, only the first has to be taken. Then all else follows. The first is the last, if you understand. The beginning is the end; the alpha *is* the omega.

The second question:

*Please describe the developmental gap between the man of spiritual experience who has already attained a certain degree of higher awareness, even certain psychic skills and capacities, and the fully enlightened being — the living Buddha.*

This is the difference: a man who has become absolutely positive is the man of spiritual attainment. The person who has become absolutely negative. . . When I say absolutely negative, I mean ninety-nine percent negative, because absolute negativity is not possible. Neither absolute positivity is possible. The other is needed. The quantity can change; the degrees differ.

The man who is ninety-nine percent negative and one percent positive is the most fallen man, what Christians call the sinner — one percent positive! That too is needed only to help his ninety-nine percent negativity. But in everything negative, whatsoever you say, only no is the response. Whatsoever existence asks, only no is the response. The atheist who cannot say yes to anything, who has become incapable of saying yes, who cannot trust — this man suffers hell. And because he says no to everything, he becomes a no, a yawning no; anger, violence, suppression, sadness, all together — he becomes a hell personified.

Difficult to find such a man because it is difficult to be such a man. To live in ninety-nine percent hell is very difficult. But just to explain to you, I am telling this. This is the mathematical possibility. One can become if one tries. You will not find such a man anywhere. Even a Hitler is not that destructive. The whole energy becomes destructive — not only of others, but of oneself also. The whole attitude is suicidal. When a person commits suicide what he is saying? He is saying no to life through his death. He is saying no to God, that "You cannot create me. I will destroy myself."

Sartre, one of the great thinkers of this age, says that suicide is the only freedom — freedom from God. Why freedom from God? Because there is no freedom. You don't have any freedom to create yourself. Whenever you are, you find yourself already created. Birth you cannot take: that is not your freedom. Sartre says, "But death you can commit; that is your freedom." You can say at least one thing definitively to God — that "I am free". This man who lives always near the abyss of suicide is the last, the greatest sinner.

In existentialism, which Sartre preaches, these words have become very meaningful — anguish, boredom, sadness. They have to become meaningful because this man will live in anguish, boredom. One percent positive is needed. He will say yes to boredom, to suicide, to anguish, only for this much: he has a need to say yes. This is the modern man who is coming nearer and nearer to this last shore. On the other peak exists the spiritual man. This is the sinner, the fallen. On the other peak — ninety-nine percent positive, one percent negative — is the spiritual man. He says yes to everything. He has only one no and that no is against no, that's all. Otherwise he is yes. But because total yes cannot exist, he has a need to say no.

This man attains many things because the positive mind can give you millions of things: this man will be happy, serene, collected, calm and quiet. And because of this the mind will flower and give all its positive qualities to him. He will have certain powers. He can read your thoughts, he can heal you. His blessing will become a force. Just by being near him, you will be benefited. In subtle ways, he is a blessing.

All the *siddhis* — all the powers that yoga talks, and

Patanjali will talk later on — will be easy to him; he will be a man of miracles, his touch will be magical. Anything is possible because he has a ninety-nine percent positive mind. Positivity is a force, a power. He will be very powerful. But still he is not enlightened. And it will be easier for you to think this man that he is enlightened than to think an enlightened man as enlightened, because the enlightened man simply goes beyond you. You cannot understand him; he becomes incomprehensible.

In fact an enlightened man has no power because he has no mind. He is not miraculous. He has no mind; he cannot do anything. He is the ultimate in non-doing. Miracles can happen around him. But they happen because of your mind, not because of him, and that is the difference. A spiritual man can do miracles; an enlightened man no. Miracles are possible, but they will happen because of you, not because of him. Your trust, your faith, will do the miracle, because you become the positive mind in that moment.

Jesus says: a woman touched his gown; he was moving in a crowd, and the woman was so poor and so old she never could believe that Jesus will bless her. So she thought it will be good to be in the crowd, and when Jesus passes, just to touch his gown. "It is *his* gown, and the very touch is enough. And I am so poor and so old, who will take care of me, who will bother? There will be many people, and Jesus will be interested in them." So she simply touched the garb.

Jesus looked back, and the woman said, "I am healed." Jesus said, "It is because of your faith. I have not done anything: you have done to yourself."

Many miracles can happen, but the man who is enlightened cannot do anything. Mind is the doer — doer of all. When mind is not there, happenings are there but no more doings. An enlightened man, in fact, is no more. He exists as a non-entity, as an emptiness. He is a shrine — empty. You can enter in him, but you will not meet him. He has gone beyond the polarities; he is a great beyond. You will be lost in him, but you cannot find him.

A man of spiritual powers is still in the world. He is your polar opposite. You feel helpless; he feels powerful. You feel unhealthy; he can heal you. It is bound to be so. You are ninety-nine percent negative; he is ninety-nine percent positive. The very meeting is between impotence and power. Positivity is power; negativity is impotence. And you will be very much impressed by such a man, and that becomes the danger for him. The more you are impressed by him, the more ego strengthens. With a negative man, the ego cannot be very much because ego needs positive power.

That's why, in sinners, you can find very, very humble people, but never in saints. Saints are always egotistic. They are somebody — powerful, chosen, elite, messengers of God, prophets. They are somebody. A sinner is humble — afraid of himself, moves carefully; he knows who he is. It has happened many times that a sinner has taken a direct jump and has become enlightened, but it has never been so easy for a man of spiritual power because the very power becomes the hindrance.

Patanjali will talk much about it. He has a complete section of these sutras devoted to *vibhuti pada* — to this dimension of power. And he has written the whole part just to make you beware that don't become a victim of it, because ego is very subtle. It is such a subtle phenomenon and such a deceptive force, and wherever there is power it sucks on it. It is a sucking phenomenon, this ego. So in the world the ego finds politics, prestige, power, wealth. Then it feels somebody — you are a president of a country or a prime minister: then you are somebody. Or you have millions of rupees — then you are somebody: ego is strengthened.

The game remains the same because the positive is

not out of the world. The positive is within the world —
better than the negative, but then the danger is also
more, because a man who feels himself very great because he is a prime minister or a president or a very rich
man he also knows that he cannot carry these riches
beyond death. But a man who feels powerful because of
psychic forces — ESP, thought-reading, clairvoyance,
clair-audience, astral traveling, healing — he feels more
egoistic. He knows he can carry these powers beyond
death. And, yes, they can be carried, because it is mind
who is reborn, and these forces belong to the mind.

Wealth belongs to the body, not to the mind: you
cannot carry it. A political power belongs to the body —
when you are dead, you are nobody. But these forces,
these spiritual powers, belong to the mind, and the mind
moves from one body to another. It is carried. You will
be born in next life as a charismatic child from the very
beginning, you will have a magnetic force in you.
Hence, more attraction; hence, more danger.

Remember, don't try to become spiritual. Spiritual is
against material just as negative, positive. In fact, they
are not opposites. The quality of both is the same. One
is superior and subtle; another is gross and inferior, but
both are the same. Don't be deceived by spiritual powers. And whenever spiritual powers start arising in you,
you have to be more alert than ever. And they will
arise! The more you will meditate, the mind will become
refined. And when the mind is refined, seeds which you
have been carrying always start sprouting. Now the soil
is ready and the season has come. And beautiful are
those flowers. . .

When you can touch somebody and heal immediately, it is difficult to resist the temptation. When you can
do much benefit to people, you can become a great
servant; it is very difficult to resist the temptation, and
immediately temptations arise and you rationalize because this is just for the service of the people that you

are doing it. But look within: through the service of the people the ego is arising, and now the greatest barrier will be there.

Materialism is not such a great barrier. It is just like the negative mind—not a great barrier to drop. It is suffering. Positive is difficult to drop, spirituality is difficult to drop. You can drop the body easily: to drop the mind is the real problem. But unless you drop both the material and the spiritual—neither this nor that—unless you go beyond both, you are not enlightened.

A man who is enlightened in fact becomes simply very, very ordinary. He has nothing special, and that is the specialty. He is so ordinary that you can bypass him on the street. You cannot bypass a spiritual man. He will bring a wave around him; he will be energy. You will be simply bathed by him if he passes you on the road—attracted like a magnet.

But you can pass a Buddha. If you don't know that he is a Buddha, you will not know. But you cannot pass a Rasputin. And Rasputin is not a bad man: Rasputin is a spiritual man. You cannot pass a Rasputin. The moment you see him, you are magnetized. You will follow him your whole life. This happened to the Csar. Once he saw this man he became a slave to him. He had a tremendous power. He will come like a strong wind; it is difficult not to be attracted by him.

It is difficult to be attracted to a Buddha. Many times you can bypass him. He is so simple and so ordinary, and that is the extraordinariness, because now the negative, positive are both lost. He is no more under the electric realm. He exists! He exists like a rock, like a tree. He exists like a sky. If you allow him, he can enter in you; he will not even knock at your door—no!—he will not be even that much aggressive. He is a very very silent phenomenon; he is a nothingness.

But this is the greatest thing to achieve because only he knows what existence is, only he knows what being is. With the negative and the positive you know the mind: negative is impotent, positive is powerful. Never try to be spiritual—it will happen automatically, you need not try it. And when it happens, remain detached.

There are many, many stories in the past. Buddha had a cousin-brother: Devadatta was his name. He took initiation from Buddha. He was a cousin-brother and of course, deep down, jealous—and very powerful man like Rasputin. Soon he started gathering his own following, and he started telling people that "I can do many things and this Buddha cannot do anything."

Followers again and again came to Buddha and said that "This Devadatta is trying to create a separate sect, and he says that he is more powerful." And he was right, but his power belonged to the positive mind. He made many efforts to kill Buddha. He made an elephant mad. When I say he made an elephant mad, I mean that he used his positive power, and it was such a strong phenomenon the elephant became intoxicated. He rushed madly; he tore down many trees. Devadatta was very happy because just behind the trees was sitting Buddha, and the elephant was going mad—just a mad energy. But when the elephant came near Buddha, he looked at the Buddha—sat silently in deep meditation, that elephant. . . Devadatta was puzzled.

What happened? When there is emptiness, everything is absorbed. Emptiness has no limits to it. The madness was absorbed. Not that Buddha has done anything—he has not done anything—he is just a vacuum. The elephant came and lost his energy, became silent. He became so silent that it is said Devadatta tried many times, but again he could not make that elephant mad.

The enlightened man is not a man at all—one thing. He is not at all—another thing. He appears to be there but he is not. You see his body but not him. The more you search him, the less is the possibility to find him. In the very search you will be lost. He has become the universal. The spiritual man is still an individual.

So remember, your mind will try to become spiritual. Your mind has a hankering to be more powerful, to be somebody in this world of nobodies. Be alert of it. Even if much benefit can be done through it, it is dangerous; the benefit is only on the surface. Deep down you are killing yourself, and soon it will be lost and again you will fall into the negative. It is a certain energy. You can lose it; you can make use of it; then it is gone.

Hindus have a very scientific category; nowhere exists that categorization. In the West they think in terms of hell and heaven — just two things. Hindus think in three categories — hell, heaven and *moksha*. It is difficult to translate the third into western languages because there exists no category. We call it liberation, but it is not. It gives the feeling, the fragrance of it just, but not exactly the same.

Heaven and hell, they are there. The third is not there. Hell is negative mind in its perfection; heaven is positive mind in its perfection. But where is the beyond? In India they say if you are a spiritualist, when you will die you will be born in a heaven. You will live there for millions of years happy, absolutely enjoying everything — but then you will have to fall back to the earth again. Energy lost, you will have to come back. You earned a particular energy, then you used it. You will fall back again to the same situation.

So they said don't seek heaven in India. Even if for millions of years you will be happy, that happy is not going to be forever. You will lose it, you will fall back; it is not worth the effort. What Hindus call *devatas* — those who live in heaven, the people who reside in heaven. . .

They are not *muktas:* they are not enlightened. But they are positive; they have reached to the peak of their positive energy, the mind energy. They can fly in the sky; they can move from one point of space to another immediately with no time gap. The moment they desire something, immediately it is fulfilled with no time gap. Here you desire, there it is fulfilled. They have beautiful, ever-young bodies. They become never old. Their bodies are golden. They live in golden cities with young women, with wine and women and dancing, and they are continuously happy. In fact, only one trouble exists there—that is boredom; they get bored. That is the only negative—one percent negative, ninety-nine percent they are happy—simply they get bored, and sometimes even they try to come on the earth. They can come; they come and they try to mingle with human beings just to get out of the boredom.

But finally they fall back. . .as if finally you come out of a dream, a beautiful dream, that's all. Heaven is a dream according to Hindus—beautiful dream. Hell is also a dream—a nightmare. But both are dreams because both belong to the mind. Remember this definition: all that belongs to the mind is a dream. Positive, negative, whatsoever: mind *is* dream. To go beyond the dream, to awake, is to become enlightened.

Difficult to say anything about the enlightened man, because he cannot be defined. Definition is possible if there is some limitation. He is vast as a sky; definition is not possible. The only way to know an enlightened man is to become enlightened. The spiritual man can be defined; he has his limitations. Within the mind, there is no difficulty in defining him.

When we will come to *vibhuti pada*—to Patanjali's sutras about *siddhis*, powers, we will see he can be defined completely. And in the West, scientific research is going on which they call psychic research. Psychic societies exist all over the world; many universities now have labs for psychic research. Sooner or later, what Patanjali says will be scientifically categorized and proved.

In a way it is good. It is good because then you will

be able to know that this is something of the mind which can be even examined by mechanical devices, categorized and finished. You cannot have any glimpse through any mechanical device of enlightenment. It is not a phenomenon of the body or of the mind. It is very elusive, mysterious.

Remember one thing: never try to gain any spiritual powers. Even if they come on your path by themselves, drop them as immediately as possible. Don't move in their company and don't listen to their tricks. They will say that "What is wrong in it? You can help others; you can become a great benefactor." But don't become that. You say simply that "I am not in search of power and nobody can help anybody." You can become an entertainment but you cannot help anybody.

And how can you help anybody? Everybody moves according to his own karmas. In fact, if a man of spiritual power touches you and your disease disappears, what is happening? Deep down your disease was to disappear; your karmas were fulfilled. It is just an excuse that it disappeared by the touch of a spiritual man. It was to disappear: because you did something, that's why it was there. The time has come. . .

You cannot help anybody in any way. There is only one help, and that is you become that which you would like everybody to become. You simply become that. Your very presence, not your doing, will be helpful.

What Buddha does? He is simply there, available, like a river. Those who are thirsty, they come. Even if a river tries to satisfy your thirst, it is impossible if you are not ready. If you don't open your mouth, if you don't bow down to receive the water, even a river may be flowing, you can remain thirsty. And this is what is happening: the river is flowing and you are sitting on the bank thirsty. The ego will always remain thirsty, whatsoever it attains. Ego is thirst. Satiety is of the soul, not of the ego.

The third question:

*What is the secret of how you can work on so many of us at the same time?*

Because I don't work at all! I am simply there; it doesn't make any difference how many are around me. If I work, then, of course, how can I work on so many at the same time? My work is of a different quality. It is not, in fact, work. I have to use these words because of you. I am simply here; things will happen if you are also here. I am available; if you are also available, things will happen by themselves; nothing is needed to be done.

A meeting is needed of two availabilities, of two presences; then things happen by themselves. What you do when you put a seed in the earth? What you do? There is just the meeting of the seed and the earth, and things happen by themselves, just like that.

I am here. If you are also here. . .and that is the problem: you may seem to be here and you may not be here. Then nothing happens. I am here. If you are also here, things happen by themselves — just like that; I am not doing anything, otherwise, I will get tired of you. I am never tired because I am not doing anything. You cannot tire me; I am not bored — otherwise, I will be bored. Even you are bored with yourselves — so many of you.

It happened in a Jewish community: a rabbi threatened to leave, and the holy days were coming near and the trustees were worried what to do. It is difficult now, at this moment, to find a rabbi, a new rabbi, and he was adamant — the old one. So they tried to persuade him; they sent a delegation of three trustees, and they told the trustees to persuade anyhow. If he wants more salary, say okay, or tell him: "At least for few weeks be here and then you can leave; then we will be able to find." So they went, and they persuaded and they tried in every

way. And they said that "We love you and we respect
you. Why are you leaving?" The rabbi said that "If
only five persons were like you here, I would have
remained!"

They felt flattered because he had said, "If only five
persons were like you here, I would have remained."
They felt very good and they said, "But it will not be
very difficult: three we are here; two more can be
found." The rabbi said, "It is not difficult; that is the
problem. There are like you two hundred persons here,
and it is too much!"

You are bored with yourself. Look in the mirror: you
are bored with your face. And so many of you are here,
I must be bored to death! And the same problems you
go on bringing to me every day. But I am never bored
because I am not working. This is not a work at all. You
may call it a love, but not a work — and love is never
bored. Thousand times you can bring the same problems to me — again and again. . .and there are not many
problems.

I have been watching thousands of people. The same
problems repeat again and again. Your problems are
just like seven days of the week — not more than that.
Again comes the Monday, again comes the Tuesday: it
goes on and on. But I am not bored a little bit because I
am not working. If you are working, then of course it is
very very difficult. That's why I can work — because I
am not working.

On so many of you, the only thing required is from
you, not from me. So you may be tired someday of me;
that's possible. You may try to escape from me; that's
possible. Only one thing is required of you. If you can
do that, then there is no need to do anything either on
my part or on your part. And that thing is your availability: you be here and now, and then it makes no difference whether you are here in this city, in this ashram, or
to the other corner of the world.

If you are available, the seeds will sprout. I am available everywhere: that is not the point. Even when I am not in this body, I will be available. But it will be more and more difficult for you, because you are not available even when I am in this body here and now just talking to you — but you are not listening. You are hearing of course, but not listening. You are looking at me, but not at me. Look at me! It is not a work! It is just a love available, and through love everything is possible — every transformation.

The fourth question:

*You mentioned that love is a need. Why is this essential need always so hard to fulfill for most people?*

Many things are involved. One thing: society is against love because love is a greatest bond, and love separates you from the society. Two lovers become a world in themselves; they don't bother about anybody. Hence, society is against; society doesn't want you to love. Marriage — granted; but not love, because once you love a person you become a world in yourself, separate. You don't bother what is happening in the world to others; you simply forget them. You create a private world of your own.

Love is such a creative force, it becomes a universe. Then you start moving around your own center — and this society cannot tolerate. Your parents cannot tolerate your love because if you are in love you forget them completely, as if they never existed. Then they exist on the margin, somewhere very distant. How can they allow you to love? They will make arrangements for your marriage. That will be their arrangement. You will exist. . .as part of the family.

Mulla Nasruddin fell in love with a woman. He came very happy home and when they were taking their supper he told the family that "I have decided." The father immediately said, "This is not possible. Impossible! — I cannot allow it because the family of the girl has not left a single *paisa* for her. She is bankrupt. Better girls are available with better dowries. Don't be foolish."

The mother said, "That girl? We never could imagine that you can be such a stupid. Because she never does anything except in reading silly novels. She is of no use. She cannot cook; she cannot clean the house. Look at the dirty house she lives in."

And so on, so forth. Every member rejected according to his own conception. The younger brother says, "I am not agreeing because of her nose. The nose is so ugly." And everybody had his opinion.

Then Nasruddin said, "But one thing that girl has which we don't have." They all asked in a chorus, "What is that?" He said, "The family: she doesn't have the family. That is one thing beautiful about her."

Parents will be against love. They will train you from the very beginning — train you in such a way that you don't fall in love, because love will go against family, and the society is nothing but a greater family. Love goes against society, civilization, religion, priests. Love is such an involvement, such a total commitment, it goes against everybody. And everybody has an investment in you.

No, it cannot be allowed. You have been trained not to love — that's the difficulty. This difficulty comes from the society, culture, civilization, all that is around you, but this is not the greatest difficulty. There is still one that comes from you and which is even greater, and that is: love needs a surrender; love needs that you should drop the ego.

And you are also against love. You would like love to become a celebration of your ego; you would like love to become an ornament for your ego. You would like love to follow you like a dog, but love never follows anybody like a dog. Love needs you in a total surrender. It is not that the woman surrenders to the man or that the man surrenders to the woman — no! Both surrender to love. Love is a god; love is really the only god, and it requires you, both the lovers, to be completely surrendered to it.

And lovers — what they are doing? The husband tries that the wife should surrender to him and the wife tries the husband should surrender to her. How can love be possible? Love is something else — both should surrender to it, and both should disappear into it.

This becomes the greatest barrier: you cannot love because of you. These two things together and love becomes impossible: and if love becomes impossible, life becomes impossible. If love becomes impossible, prayer becomes impossible. If love becomes impossible, God becomes impossible. All that is beautiful grows out of love. The soil of love is a must; otherwise you will remain crippled. And then you try to complement and supplement it in other ways, but nothing can supplement it. No substitute exists.

You can go on doing prayer, but your prayer will lack the grace that comes when one has loved. How can you *do* prayer? Your prayer will be just rubbish — a verbal phenomenon. You will say something to God and talk to him and go to sleep, but it will lack the essential quality. How can you pray when you have not loved? Prayer comes through the heart — and your heart has remained closed, so prayer comes from the head, and head cannot become the heart.

So all over the world, people go on praying. They are just gestures; the essential is not there. The prayer is without roots. Love prepares the soil. It prepares the ground for the prayer to come. Prayer is nothing but a higher love — a love which transcends individuals, a love which goes to the whole, not to the part. But you need learning with the part.

You cannot just jump into the ocean. Learn swimming in a swimming pool. Love is a swimming pool where you are protected and you can learn; then you can go to the seas, to the wild seas. You cannot take the jump into the wild seas directly — if you take, you will be in danger — that's not possible. Love is a small swimming pool — two persons only: the whole world very small. . .possible to enter into each other.

Even there you are afraid. In a swimming pool you are afraid that "I may be gone, drowned." Then what to say about ocean? Love is the first grounding, the first readiness to take a greater jump. I teach you love, and I tell you that whatsoever is at stake, don't bother: sacrifice it, whatsoever — prestige, wealth, family, society, culture — whatsoever is at stake, don't bother. Be a gambler because there is nothing like love. If you lose everything, you lose nothing if you gain love. If you lose love, whatsoever you gain you gain nothing. And be aware: these two things.

The society will not help you; it is against. Love is an anti-social force, and the society tries to suppress love; then you can be used in many ways. For example, if you are really in love, you cannot be made a soldier; you cannot be sent to the war. Impossible because you don't bother. . . You say, "What is a country? What is this patriotism? Nonsense!" Love is such a beautiful flower; one who has known — patriotism, nationalism, country, the flag, all look nonsense. You have tasted the real thing.

The society tries to divert. The real thing should not be tasted. Then you are hankering for love, and your love can be diverted to any direction. It can become patriotism; then you can go and become a martyr. You are a fool, because you are wasting yourself! You can go and die; your love has been diverted. If you don't love, your love can become love of money. Then you become an accumulator, hoarder. Then your family is happy — you are doing beautifully.

You are simply committing suicide. The family is happy because you are accumulating so much wealth. They missed their life; now they are forcing you to miss your life. And they do it in such a loving way that you cannot say no also. They make you feel guilty. If you hoard money they are happy. But how a man who loves can hoard? Difficult; a lover is never a hoarder. A lover shares, distributes, goes on giving; a lover cannot hoard.

When love is not there, you become miserly because you are afraid. You don't have the shelter of love, so you need some shelter. Wealth becomes the substitute. The society also wants you to hoard, because how wealth is to be created if everyone becomes a lover? The society will be very, very rich, but rich in a totally different way. It may be poor materially, but it will be rich spiritually.

But that richness is not visible. The society needs visible wealth, so in the whole world, religion, society, culture, they are in a conspiracy because you have only one energy: that is love energy. If it moves rightly into love, then it cannot be forced to move anywhere else. If you don't love, your very missing of love may become a research into science.

Freud had many glimpses of truth. He was really a rare man; so many insights happened to him. He said whenever you penetrate anything, it is penetrating the woman, and if you are not allowed the woman, you will try to penetrate something else. You may penetrate toward being a prime minister of a country.

Politicians you will never find lovers: they will always sacrifice love for their power. Scientists will never be lovers, because if they become lovers they relax. They need a tension, a constant obsession. Love relaxes; constant obsession is not possible. They go madly to their laboratory. They are obsessed, possessed. Night and day they work.

History knows that whenever a country's love-need

is fulfilled, the country becomes weak. Then it can be defeated. So the love-need should not be fulfilled. Then the country is dangerous because everybody is a maniac and ready to fight. For slightest provocation, everybody is ready to fight. If love-need is fulfilled, then who bothers! Just think, if really the whole country has been in love, and somebody attacks. . .we will say to them, "Okay, you also come and be here. Why bother? We are so happy — you also come, and the country is vast; you also be here and be happy. And if you want to be the rulers, be the rulers — nothing is wrong; so far so good. You take the responsibility — good!"

But when love-need is not fulfilled, you are always ready to fight. You just remember. Just try to watch your own mind. If you have not loved your woman for few days, you are constantly irritated. You love and you relax. Irritation goes, and you feel so good — you can forgive. A lover can forgive everything. Love has been such a blessing, he can forgive all that is wrong.

No, leaders won't allow you to love because then soldiers cannot be created. Then where you will find warmongers, maniacs, mad people who would like to destroy? Love is creativity. If love-need is fulfilled, you would like to create, not to destroy. Then the whole political structure will fall down. If you love, then the whole family structure will be totally different. If you love, then the economy and the economics will be different. In fact, if love is allowed, the whole world will take a totally different shape. It cannot be allowed because this structure has its investments. Every structure pushes itself onward, and if you are crushed it doesn't bother.

Whole humanity is crushed, and the chariot of civilization goes on and on. Realize this, watch this, be aware of this — and then love is so simple; nothing is more simple than that. Drop all that society needs; remember your inner needs. That is not going against society. You are simply trying to enrich your own life. You are not here to fulfill anybody else's expectations. You are here for your thing—for your own fulfillment.

Make that the primary, the base, and don't bother about other things. Because mad people are all around you, they will push you toward madness. No need to go against the society; just drop out of its investments, that's all.

You need not become rebellious, a revolutionary, because that too again is coming to the same thing. If your love is not fulfilled, you will become a revolutionary, because that too is a destruction in garb. And then comes the real problem: drop your own ego. Love needs total surrender.

Allow this to happen, because there is nothing else which can happen to you. You will be wasted if you don't allow it to happen. And if you allow it to happen, many more things become possible. One thing leads to another. Love always leads to prayer. That's why Jesus insists God is love.

# BOOKS PUBLISHED BY
# RAJNEESH FOUNDATION
# INTERNATIONAL

For a complete catalog of all the books published by
Rajneesh Foundation International, contact:

Rajneesh Foundation International
P.O. Box 9
Rajneeshpuram, Oregon 97741 USA
(503) 489-3462

## THE BAULS

The Beloved (2 volumes)

## BUDDHA

The Book of the Books (volume 1 & 2)
*the Dhammapada*

The Diamond Sutra
*the Vajrachchedika Prajnaparamita Sutra*

The Discipline of Transcendence (4 volumes)
*the Sutra of 42 Chapters*

The Heart Sutra
*the Prajnaparamita Hridayam Sutra*

## BUDDHIST MASTERS

The Book of Wisdom (volume 1)
*Atisha's Seven Points of Mind Training*

The White Lotus
*the sayings of Bodhidharma*

## EARLY DISCOURSES

And Now, and Here (volume 1)

Beware of Socialism

The Long and the Short and the All

The Perfect Way

## HASSIDISM

The Art of Dying

The True Sage

## JESUS

Come Follow Me (4 volumes)
*the sayings of Jesus*

I Say Unto You (2 volumes)
*the sayings of Jesus*

## KABIR

The Divine Melody

Ecstasy: The Forgotten Language

The Fish in the Sea is Not Thirsty

The Guest

The Path of Love

The Revolution

## RESPONSES TO QUESTIONS

Be Still and Know

From Sex to Superconsciousness

The Goose is Out

My Way: The Way of the White Clouds

Walking in Zen, Sitting in Zen

Walk Without Feet, Fly Without Wings
and Think Without Mind

Zen: Zest, Zip, Zap and Zing

## SUFISM

Just Like That

The Perfect Master (2 volumes)

The Secret

Sufis: The People of the Path (2 volumes)

Unio Mystica (2 volumes)
*the Hadiqa of Hakim Sanai*

Until You Die

The Wisdom of the Sands (2 volumes)

## TANTRA

The Book of the Secrets (volumes 4 & 5)
*Vigyana Bhairava Tantra*

Tantra, Spirituality & Sex
*Excerpts from The Book of the Secrets*

Tantra: The Supreme Understanding
*(Tilopa's Song of Mahamudra)*

The Tantra Vision (2 volumes)
*the Royal Song of Saraha*

## TAO

The Empty Boat
*the stories of Chuang Tzu*

The Secret of Secrets (2 volumes)
*the Secret of the Golden Flower*

Tao: The Golden Gate (volume 1)

Tao: The Pathless Path (2 volumes)
*the stories of Lieh Tzu*

Tao: The Three Treasures (4 volumes)
*the Tao Te Ching of Lao Tzu*

When The Shoe Fits
*the stories of Chuang Tzu*

## THE UPANISHADS

I Am That
*(Isa Upanishad)*

The Ultimate Alchemy (2 volumes)
*Atma Pooja Upanishad*

Vedanta: Seven Steps to Samadhi
*Akshya Upanishad*

Philosophia Ultima
*Mandukya Upanishad*

## WESTERN MYSTICS

The Hidden Harmony
*the fragments of Heraclitus*

The New Alchemy: To Turn You On
*Mabel Collins' Light on the Path*

# INITIATION TALKS
## between Master disciple

Hammer On The Rock
*(December 10, 1975 - January 15, 1976)*

Above All Don't Wobble
*(January 16 - February 12, 1976)*

Nothing To Lose But Your Head
*(February 13 - March 12, 1976)*

Be Realistic: Plan For a Miracle
*(March 13 - April 6, 1976)*

Get Out of Your Own Way
*(April 7 - May 2, 1976)*

Beloved of My Heart
*(May 3 - 28, 1976)*

The Cypress in the Courtyard
*(May 29 - June 27, 1976)*

A Rose is a Rose is a Rose
*(June 28 - July 27, 1976)*

Dance Your Way to God
*(July 28 - August 20, 1976)*

The Passion for the Impossible
*(August 21 - September 18, 1976)*

The Great Nothing
*(September 19 - October 11, 1976)*

God is Not for Sale
*(October 12 - November 7, 1976)*

The Shadow of the Whip
*(November 8 - December 3, 1976)*

Blessed are the Ignorant
*(December 4 - 31, 1976)*

The Buddha Disease
*(January 1977)*

What Is, Is, What Ain't, Ain't
*(February 1977)*

The Zero Experience
*(March 1977)*

For Madmen Only (Price of Admission: Your Mind)
*(April 1977)*

This Is It
*(May 1977)*

The Further Shore
*(June 1977)*

Far Beyond the Stars
*(July 1977)*

The No Book (No Buddha, No Teaching, No Discipline)
*(August 1977)*

Don't Just Do Something, Sit There
*(September 1977)*

Only Losers Can Win in this Game
*(October 1977)*

The Open Secret
*(November 1977)*

The Open Door
*(December 1977)*

The Sun Behind the Sun Behind the Sun
*(January 1978)*

Believing the Impossible Before Breakfast
*(February 1978)*

Don't Bite My Finger, Look Where I am Pointing
*(March 1978)*

Let Go!
*(April 1978)*

The Ninety-Nine Names of Nothingness
*(May 1978)*

The Madman's Guide to Enlightenment
*(June 1978)*

Don't Look Before You Leap
*(July 1978)*

Hallelujah!
*(August 1978)*

God's Got a Thing About You
*(September 1978)*

The Tongue-Tip Taste of Tao
*(October 1978)*

The Sacred Yes
*(November 1978)*

Turn On, Tune In, and Drop the Lot
*(December 1978)*

Zorba the Buddha
*(January 1979)*

Won't You Join the Dance?
*(February 1979)*

You Ain't Seen Nothin' Yet
*(March 1979)*

The Shadow of the Bamboo
*(April 1979)*

The Sound of One Hand Clapping
*(March 1981)*

OTHER TITLES

The Book
*an introduction to the teachings of*
 *Bhagwan Shree Rajneesh*
 *Series I from A to H*
 *Series II from I to Q*
 *Series III from R to Z*

A Cup of Tea
*letters to disciples*

The Orange Book
*the meditation techniques of*
 *Bhagwan Shree Rajneesh*

Rajneeshism
*an introduction to Bhagwan Shree Rajneesh and His*
 *religion*

The Sound of Running Water
*a photobiography of*
 *Bhagwan Shree Rajneesh and His work, 1974-1978*

This Very Place The Lotus Paradise
*a photobiography of*
  *Bhagwan Shree Rajneesh and His work, 1978-1984*

## BOOKS FROM OTHER PUBLISHERS

## ENGLISH EDITIONS
### UNITED KINGDOM

The Art of Dying
*(Sheldon Press)*

The Book of the Secrets (volume 1)
*(Thames & Hudson)*

Dimensions Beyond the Known
*(Sheldon Press)*

The Hidden Harmony
*(Sheldon Press)*

Meditation: The Art of Ecstasy
*(Sheldon Press)*

The Mustard Seed
*(Sheldon Press)*

Neither This Nor That
*(Sheldon Press)*

No Water, No Moon
*(Sheldon Press)*

Roots and Wings
*(Routledge & Kegan Paul)*

Straight to Freedom (Original title:
Until You Die)
*(Sheldon Press)*

The Supreme Doctrine
*(Routledge & Kegan Paul)*

The Supreme Understanding (Original title:
Tantra: The Supreme Understanding)
*(Sheldon Press)*

Tao: The Three Treasures (volume 1)
*(Wildwood House)*

# UNITED STATES OF AMERICA

The Book of the Secrets (volumes 1-3)
*(Harper & Row)*

The Great Challenge
*(Grove Press)*

Hammer on the Rock
*(Grove Press)*

I Am The Gate
*(Harper & Row)*

Journey Toward the Heart (Original title:
Until You Die)
*(Harper & Row)*

Meditation: The Art of Ecstasy
*(Harper & Row)*

The Mustard Seed
*(Harper & Row)*

My Way: The Way of the White Clouds
*(Grove Press)*

Only One Sky (Original title:
Tantra: The Supreme Understanding)
*(Dutton)*

The Psychology of the Esoteric
*(Harper & Row)*

Roots and Wings
*(Routledge & Kegan Paul)*

The Supreme Doctrine
*(Routledge & Kegan Paul)*

Words Like Fire (Original title:
Come Follow Me, volume 1)
*(Harper & Row)*

**BOOKS ON BHAGWAN**

The Awakened One: The Life and Work
of Bhagwan Shree Rajneesh
*by Swami Satya Vedant*
*(Harper & Row)*

Death Comes Dancing: Celebrating Life
with Bhagwan Shree Rajneesh
*by Ma Satya Bharti*
*(Routledge & Kegan Paul)*

Drunk On The Divine
*by Ma Satya Bharti*
*(Grove Press)*

The Ultimate Risk
*by Ma Satya Bharti*
*(Routledge & Kegan Paul)*

Dying For Enlightenment
*by Bernard Gunther (Swami Deva Amitprem)*
*(Harper & Row)*

Neo-Tantra
*by Bernard Gunther (Swami Deva Amitprem)*
*(Harper & Row)*

## FOREIGN LANGUAGE EDITIONS
## DANISH

### TRANSLATIONS

Hemmelighedernes Bog (volume 1)
*(Borgens Forlag)*

Hu-Meditation Og Kosmisk Orgasme
*(Borgens Forlag)*

### BOOKS ON BHAGWAN

Sjælens Oprør
*by Swami Deva Satyarthi*
*(Borgens Forlag)*

## DUTCH

### TRANSLATIONS

Drink Mij
*(Ankh-Hermes)*

Het Boek Der Geheimen (volumes 1-5)
*(Mirananda)*

Geen Water, Geen Maan
*(Mirananda)*

Gezaaid In Goede Aarde
*(Ankh-Hermes)*

Ik Ben De Poort
*(Ankh-Hermes)*

Ik Ben De Zee Die Je Zoekt
*(Ankh-Hermes)*

Meditatie: De Kunst van Innerlijke Extase
*(Mirananda)*

Mijn Weg, De Weg van de Witte Wolk
*(Arcanum)*

Het Mosterdzaad (volumes 1 & 2)
*(Mirananda)*

Het Oranje Meditatieboek
*(Ankh-Hermes)*

Psychologie en Evolutie
*(Ankh-Hermes)*

Tantra: Het Allerhoogste Inzicht
*(Ankh-Hermes)*

Tantra, Spiritualiteit en Seks
*(Ankh-Hermes)*

De Tantra Visie (volume 1)
*(Arcanum)*

Tau
*(Ankh-Hermes)*

Totdat Je Sterft
*(Ankh-Hermes)*

De Verborgen Harmonie
*(Mirananda)*

Volg Mij
*(Ankh-Hermes)*

Zoeken naar de Stier
*(Ankh-Hermes)*

**BOOKS ON BHAGWAN**

Bhagwan: Notities van Een Discipel
*by Swami Deva Amrito (Jan Foudraine)*
*(Ankh-Hermes)*

Bhagwan Shree Rajneesh: De Laatste Gok
*by Ma Satya Bharti*
*(Mirananda)*

Oorspronkelijk Gezicht,
Een Gang Naar Huis
*by Swami Deva Amrito (Jan Foudraine)*
*(Ambo)*

## FRENCH

**TRANSLATIONS**

L'éveil à la Conscience Cosmique
*(Dangles)*

Je Suis La Porte
*(EPI)*

Le Livre Des Secrets (volume 1)
*(Soleil Orange)*

La Meditation Dynamique
*(Dangles)*

## GERMAN

**TRANSLATIONS**

Auf der Suche
*(Sambuddha Verlag)*

Das Buch der Geheimnisse
*(Heyne Taschenbuch)*

Das Orangene Buch
*(Sambuddha Verlag)*

Der Freund
*(Sannyas Verlag)*

Sprung ins Unbekannte
*(Sannyas Verlag)*

Ekstase: Die vergessene Sprache
*(Herzschlag Verlag, formerly Ki-Buch)*

Esoterische Psychologie
*(Sannyas Verlag)*

Rebellion der Seele
*(Sannyas Verlag)*

Ich bin der Weg
*(Rajneesh Verlag)*

Intelligenz des Herzens
*(Herzschlag Verlag, formerly Ki-Buch)*

Jesus aber schwieg
*(Sannyas Verlag)*

Jesus -der Menschensohn
*(Sannyas Verlag)*

Kein Wasser, Kein Mond
*(Herzschlag Verlag, formerly Ki-Buch)*

Komm und folge mir
*(Sannyas Verlag)*

Meditation: Die Kunst zu sich selbst zu finden
*(Heyne Verlag)*

Mein Weg: Der Weg der weissen Wolke
*(Herzschlag Verlag, formerly Ki-Buch)*

Mit Wurzeln und mit Flügeln
*(Edition Lotus)*

Nicht bevor du stirbst
*(Edition Gyandip, Switzerland)*

Die Schuhe auf dem Kopf
*(Edition Lotus)*

Das Klatschen der einen Hand
*(Edition Gyandip, Switzerland)*

Spirituelle Entwicklung
*(Fischer)*

Vom Sex zum Kosmischen Bewusstsein
*(New Age)*

Yoga: Alpha und Omega
*(Edition Gyandip, Switzerland)*

Sprengt den Fels der Unbewusstheit
*(Fischer)*

Tantra: Die höchste Einsicht
*(Sambuddha Verlag)*

Tantrische Liebeskunst
*(Sannyas Verlag)*

Die Alchemie der Verwandlung
*(Edition Lotus)*

Die verborgene Harmonie
*(Sannyas Verlag)*

Was ist Meditation?
*(Sannyas Verlag)*

Die Gans ist raus!
*(Sannyas Verlag)*

**BOOKS ON BHAGWAN**

Rajneeshismus - Bhagwan Shree Rajneesh und
seine Religion
*Eine Eiufuhrung*
*Rajneesh Foundation International*

Begegnung mit Niemand
*by Mascha Rabben (Ma Hari Chetana)*
*(Herzschlag Verlag)*

Ganz entspannt im Hier und Jetzt
*by Swami Satyananda*
*(Rowohlt)*

Im Grunde ist alles ganz einfach
*by Swami Satyananda*
*(Ullstein)*

Wagnis Orange
*by Ma Satya Bharti*
*(Fachbuchhandlung fur Psychologie)*

Wenn das Herz frei wird
*by Ma Prem Gayan (Silvie Winter)*
*(Herbig)*

Der Erwachte
*by Vasant Joshi*
*(Synthesis Verlag)*

Rajneeshpuram - Fest des Foiedeus und der Liebe
*(Sannyas Verlag)*

# GREEK

**TRANSLATION**

I Krifi Armonia (The Hidden Harmony)
*(Emmanual Rassoulis)*

## HEBREW

## ITALIAN

Il Seme della Ribellione (volumes 1-3)
*(Re Nudo)*

Tantra: La Comprensione Suprema
*(Bompiani)*

Tao: I Tre Tesori (volumes 1-3)
*(Re Nudo)*

Tecniche di Liberazione
*(La Salamandra)*

Semi di Saggezza
*(SugarCo)*

BOOKS ON BHAGWAN

Rajneeshismo
*una introduzione a
  Bhagwan Shree Rajneesh a sua religione*

Alla Ricerca del Dio Perduto
*by Swami Deva Majid
(SugarCo)*

Il Grande Esperimento:
  Meditazioni E Terapie Nell'ashram
Di Bhagwan Shree Rajneesh
*by Ma Satya Bharti
(Armenia)*

L'Incanto D'Arancio
*by Swami Swatantra Sarjano
(Savelli)*

# JAPANESE

TRANSLATIONS

Dance Your Way to God
*(Rajneesh Publications)*

The Empty Boat (volumes 1 & 2)
*(Rajneesh Publications)*

From Sex to Superconsciousness
*(Rajneesh Publications)*

The Grass Grows by Itself
*(Fumikura)*

The Heart Sutra
*(Merkmal)*

Meditation: The Art of Ecstasy
*(Merkmal)*

The Mustard Seed
*(Merkmal)*

My Way: The Way of the White Clouds
*(Rajneesh Publications)*

The Orange Book
*(Wholistic Therapy Institute)*

The Search
*(Merkmal)*

The Beloved
*(Merkmal)*

Tantra: The Supreme Understanding
*(Merkmal)*

Tao: The Three Treasures (volumes 1-4)
*(Merkmal)*

Until You Due
*(Fumikura)*

Rajneeshism
*an introduction to*
  *Bhagwan Shree Rajneesh and His religion*

## PORTUGUESE (BRAZIL)

TRANSLATIONS

O Cipreste No Jardim
*(Soma)*

Dimensões Além do Conhecido
*(Soma)*

O Livro Dos Segredos (volume 1)
*(Maha Lakshmi Editora)*

Eu Sou A Porta
*(Pensamento)*

A Harmonia Oculta
*(Pensamento)*

Meditacão: A Arte Do Extase
*(Cultrix)*

Meu Caminho:
  O Comainho Das Nuvens Brancas
*(Tao Livraria & Editora)*

Nem Agua, Nem Lua
*(Pensamento)*

O Livro Orange
*(Soma)*

Palavras De Fogo
*(Global/Ground)*

A Psicologia Do Esotérico
*(Tao Livraria & Editora)*

A Semente De Mostarda (volumes 1 & 2)
*(Tao Livraria & Editora)*

Tantra: Sexo E Espiritualidade
*(Agora)*

Tantra: A Supreme Comprensao
*(Cultrix)*

Antes Que Voce Morra
*(Maha Lakshmi Editora)*

Extase: A Linguagem Esquecida
*(Global)*

Arte de Morrer
*(Global)*

# SPANISH

TRANSLATIONS

Introducción al Mundo del Tantra
*(Colección Tantra)*

Meditación: El Arte del Extasis
*(Colección Tantra)*

Psicológia de lo Esotérico:
La Nueva Evolución del Hombre
*(Cuatro Vientos Editorial)*

¿Qué Es Meditación?
*(Koan/Roselló Impresions)*

Yo Soy La Puerta
*(Editorial Diana)*

Sòlo Un Cielo (volumes 1 & 2)
*(Colección Tantra)*

El Sutra del Corazon
*(Sarvogeet)*

Ven, Sigueme (volume 1)
*(Sagaro)*

**BOOKS ON BHAGWAN**

El Riesgo Supremo
*by Ma Satya Bharti*
*(Martinez Roca)*

SWEDISH

TRANSLATION

Den Väldiga Utmaningen
*(Livskraft)*

# RAJNEESH MEDITATION CENTERS, ASHRAMS AND COMMUNES

There are hundreds of Rajneesh meditation centers throughout the world. These are some of the main ones, which can be contacted for the name and address and telephone number of the center nearest you. They can also tell you about the availability of the books of Bhagwan Shree Rajneesh — in English or in foreign language editions. General information is available from Rajneesh Foundation International.

A wide range of meditation and inner growth programs is available throughout the year at Rajneesh International Meditation University.

For further information and a complete listing of programs, write or call:

> Rajneesh International Meditation University
> P.O. Box 5, Rajneeshpuram, OR 97741 USA
> Phone: (503) 489-3328

## USA

RAJNEESH FOUNDATION INTERNATIONAL
P.O. Box 9, Rajneeshpuram, Oregon 97741.
Tel: (503) 489-3301

UTSAVA RAJNEESH MEDITATION CENTER
20062 Laguna Canyon Rd., Laguna Beach, CA 92651.
Tel: (714) 497-4877

DEVADEEP RAJNEESH SANNYAS ASHRAM
1430 Longfellow St., N.W., Washington, D.C. 20011.
Tel: (202) 723-2188

## CANADA

ARVIND RAJNEESH SANNYAS ASHRAM
2807 W. 16th Ave., Vancouver, B.C. V6K 3C5.
Tel: (604) 734-4681

SHANTI SADAN RAJNEESH MEDITATION CENTER
P.O. Box 374, Station R, Montreal, Quebec. H2S 3M2.
Tel: (514) 272-4566

## AUSTRALIA

PREMDWEEP RAJNEESH MEDITATION CENTER
64 Fullarton Rd., Norwood, S.A. 5067. Tel: 08-423388

SATPRAKASH RAJNEESH MEDITATION CENTER
4A Ormond St., Paddington, N.S.W. 2021
Tel: (02) 336570

SAHAJAM RAJNEESH SANNYAS ASHRAM
6 Collie Street, Fremantle 6160, W.A.
Tel: (09) 336-2422

SVARUP RAJNEESH MEDITATION CENTER
303 Drummond St., Carlton 3053, Victoria. Tel: 347-3388

## BELGIUM

VADAN RAJNEESH MEDITATION CENTER
Platte-Lo-Straat 65, 3200 Leuven (Kessel-Lo).
Tel: 016/25-1487

## BRAZIL

PRASTHAN RAJNEESH MEDITATION CENTER
Caixa Postal No. 11072, Ag. Cidade Nova,
Rio de Janeiro, R.J. 20251.
Tel: 222-9476

PURNAM RAJNEESH MEDITATION CENTER
Caixa Postal 1946, Porto Alegre, RS 90000.

## CHILE

SAGARO RAJNEESH MEDITATION CENTER
Golfo de Darien 10217, Las Condes, Santiago.
Tel: 472476

## DENMARK

ANAND NIKETAN RAJNEESH MEDITATION CENTER
Stroget, Frederiksberggade 15, 1459 Copenhagen K.
Tel: (01) 139940, 117909

## EAST AFRICA

AMBHOJ RAJNEESH MEDITATION CENTER
P.O. Box 59159, Nairobi, Kenya

## GREAT BRITAIN

MEDINA RAJNEESH BODY CENTER
81 Belsize Park Gardens, London NW3.
Tel: (01) 722-8220, 722-6404

MEDINA RAJNEESH NEO-SANNYAS COMMUNE
Herringswell, Bury St. Edmunds, Suffolk 1P28 6SW.
Tel: (0638) 750234

## HOLLAND

DE STAD RAJNEESH NEO-SANNYAS COMMUNE
719 Prinsengracht, 1017 JW Amsterdam
Tel: 020-221296

## INDIA

RAJNEESHDHAM NEO-SANNYAS COMMUNE
17 Koregaon Park, Poona 411 001, MS. Tel: 28127

## ITALY

VIVEK RAJNEESH MEDITATION CENTER
Via San Marco 40/4, 20121 Milan. Tel: 659-0335

## JAPAN

SHANTIYUGA RAJNEESH MEDITATION CENTER
Sky Mansion 2F, 1-34-1 Ookayama, Meguro-ku, Tokyo 152.
Tel: (03) 724-9631

UTSAVA RAJNEESH MEDITATION CENTER
2-9-8 Hattori-Motomachi, Toyonaki-shi, Osaka 561.
Tel: 06-863-4246

## NEW ZEALAND

SHANTI NIKETAN RAJNEESH MEDITATION CENTER
119 Symonds Street, Auckland. Tel: 770-326

## PUERTO RICO

BHAGWATAM RAJNEESH MEDITATION CENTER
Box 2886, Old San Juan, PR 00905.
Tel: 765-4150

## SWEDEN

DEEVA RAJNEESH MEDITATION CENTER
Surbrunnsgatan 60, S11327 Stockholm. Tel: (08) 327788

## SWITZERLAND

KOTA RAJNEESH NEO-SANNYAS COMMUNE
Baumackerstr. 42, 8050 Zurich. Tel: (01) 312 1600

## WEST GERMANY

BAILE RAJNEESH NEO-SANNYAS COMMUNE
Karolinenstr. 7-9, 2000 Hamburg 6. Tel: (040) 432140

DORFCHEN RAJNEESH NEO-SANNYAS COMMUNE
Dahlmannstr. 9, 1000 Berlin 12. Tel: (030) 32-007-0

SATDHARMA RAJNEESH MEDITATION CENTER
Klenzestr. 41, 8000 Munich 5. Tel: (089) 269-077

WIOSKA RAJNEESH NEO-SANNYAS COMMUNE
Lutticherstr. 33/35, 5000 Cologne 1. Tel: 0221-517199

# BEWARE OF SOCIALISM

by
Bhagwan Shree Rajneesh

Five discourses given at Cross Maidan, Bombay—April 1970.

"Men are not equal. And so, if we impose equality on man with force, it will only destroy him. Man should have full opportunity to be unequal and different; he should be free to differ, to dissent, to deny, to rebel. Then only will he grow and blossom and bear fruit."

$3.95 paperback                    ISBN 0-88050-706-3

Please make payment to:
Rajneesh Foundation International
P.O. Box 9
Rajneeshpuram, OR 97741   USA